MADNESS CRACKED

MICK POWER

MADNESS
CRACKED

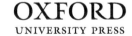
OXFORD
UNIVERSITY PRESS

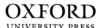

OXFORD

UNIVERSITY PRESS

Great Clarendon Street, Oxford, OX2 6DP,
United Kingdom

Oxford University Press is a department of the University of Oxford.
It furthers the University's objective of excellence in research, scholarship,
and education by publishing worldwide. Oxford is a registered trade mark of
Oxford University Press in the UK and in certain other countries

Published in the United States of America by Oxford University Press
198 Madison Avenue, New York, NY 10016, United States of America

British Library Cataloguing in Publication Data
Data available

Library of Congress Control Number: 2014947152

ISBN 978–0–19–870387–7

Printed and bound by
CPI Group (UK) Ltd, Croydon, CR0 4YY

For Charlie
—with lifelong thanks

PREFACE

Almost anything that has been said about madness, and almost any approach to what madness is, has some grain of truth in it, and every proposal that comes down on one side is guaranteed to be vehemently disagreed with by opponents from several other sides. Let us therefore consider in shorthand what some of these disputes are by beginning with the following two examples:

John believes that he is mad, but he isn't.

Tom believes that he is not mad, but he is.

These sentences summarize some of the conundrums that face any discussion or review of how we approach the question of madness. If we take a purely subjective approach to madness, John *would* be mad because he believes himself to be so, whereas by the same subjective logic Tom would *not* be mad because he does not believe himself to be so. Many practitioners working in clinical psychology might well endorse this subjective approach. For example, a client who suffers from panic attacks and believes that he is mad might well be offered a cognitive therapy intervention including challenging his beliefs about madness. Equally, a clinical psychologist working with Tom, who is hearing voices but who doesn't believe himself to be mad, might well be happy with Tom's belief and make no attempt to challenge it, while providing better coping mechanisms for managing his voices. In other words, the subjective approach to madness is alive and well and helps clients on a daily basis.

The objective approach is even more dominant and forms part of the medical model approach to madness. In this approach, John's belief that he is mad would be dismissed if on a clinical diagnostic interview none or insufficient numbers of specific symptoms were deemed to be present to warrant a diagnostic label. At least some psychiatrists would be tempted to dismiss John's belief in his "madness" as simply that of the "worried well." Equally, Tom's belief that despite hearing voices he isn't mad would be likely to be deemed a "lack of insight" and therefore one of the presenting symptoms for the objective conclusion that he exceeded the threshold on a range of symptoms in a clinical diagnostic interview.

Before anyone thinks that the problem of madness is merely that of a resolution of subjective versus objective standpoints, French philosophy, especially the provocative work of Michel Foucault, has presented an alternative middle way that cocks a snook at our simplified subjective versus objective descriptors. Again, let us take two examples in an attempt to highlight what the issues are:

> Carol believes that she is mad, society believes that she is mad, but she isn't.
>
> Jane believes that she is not mad, society believes that she is mad, but she isn't.

There are of course further possible combinations that can be added to these two examples, but the core of what they attempt to capture is the social constructionist possibility that madness is a societal construct that overrides the individual's beliefs, no matter what those beliefs are. Constructionists such as Mary Boyle (2013) would argue that the subjective approach of the clinical psychologist already outlined is wrong because it is individualistic and ignores the role of social construction, and that the objective medical model of psychiatry is pseudoscientific and reductionist because it reduces social–psychological phenomena to biological mechanisms. Stigmatization of different groups has occurred throughout history, and the "mad" represent a socially constructed stigmatized group that has been targeted in our recent industrial and post-industrial ages. However, social constructionists such as Mary Boyle miss the possibility that construction also occurs at an individual intrapsychic level because they reject the individual psychological level of explanation. Individual cognitive constructive processes (e.g., Neisser, 1976) must be considered alongside social constructive processes to cover at least the following category of possible models:

> Sergei believes that he is mad, but society believes that he is not mad.

In this example, Sergei has a personal construction that he is mad, whereas society does not believe him to be mad. Any constructionist approach to madness therefore needs to allow for inconsistent and contradictory constructions between the psychological and social levels, in addition to contradictory constructions within each level that, for example, would allow for state-dependent models of the form:

> On Mondays Victor believes he is mad, but for the rest of the week he believes that he is not mad.
>
> While anxious, Jeremy believes he is mad, but not when he is feeling happy.

The general situation represented by the subjective, the objective, and the constructionist approaches may seem as irresolvable as the conflicts between the three great monotheisms of Judaism, Christianity, and Islam. And just as pointing to the

Bible as the shared book of the three monotheisms is likely to annoy all and satisfy none, perhaps there is a meta-level at which the subjective, objective, and constructionist viewpoints all say something important about madness:

What if John's subjective belief that he is mad is important?
What if Tom's belief that he isn't mad is mistaken, that it is a false belief?
And what if society does construct stigmatized groups, of which madness is a current historical example?

That is, what if the concept of madness has to be understood as the interplay between all of these possible approaches, because no one approach is absolutely right, but equally no one approach is absolutely wrong. Each approach describes a different part of the mad elephant in the dark room, as it were.

Now tough-minded proponents of each of these three approaches will lay into such a proposal as morally and philosophically bankrupt, inconsistent, and contradictory. However, what the approach actually attempts is an integration across several levels of explanation, including the biological, the psychological, and the social, which proposes that understanding at one level cannot and should not be reduced to understanding at a lower level; nevertheless, effects permeate across the levels, though not in simple one-to-one mapping rules. Madness therefore is a construction, by the individual, by society, or by both, of a set of biopsychosocial presenting problems, but these constructions cannot simply be reduced to a set of biological signs and symptoms, in contrast to the standard medical model for physical illnesses which can be understood at a purely biomedical level. At best, the solution might be to use a "majority report" in which at least two of the systems agree on "madness" even if the third does not, as we will argue later in the book.

Let us return to Tom, who is hearing voices. A clinical diagnostic interview administered by a psychiatrist deems Tom to be suffering from schizophrenia with a lack of insight into his disorder. He is therefore prescribed medication against his will and put under section for further observation because he represents a potential danger to society. Cases such as Tom's highlight the conflict between the objective (medical model) and constructionist approaches. The stigmatization of Tom as dangerous and lacking insight leads to a social construction, which may be as inappropriate in its application to Tom as it is to the average person on the Clapham Omnibus. Social control of "madness" quite rightly becomes the focus of the conflict in such cases.

OK. Let's imagine that the Wizard of Oz has just waved his wand and we have turned into a perfectly tolerant and perfectly supportive society. There are no stigmatized groups and everyone is given the best possible care when they suffer or experience adversity. Would problems that are currently labeled as schizophrenia, psychosis, autism, or whatever simply disappear? That is, if such problems were purely social constructions, can they be deconstructed out of existence? Well, some problems may well be "treatable" in this social constructionist manner, such as in the diagnosis of "creeping" or "sluggish" schizophrenia that was used as a label for some Soviet dissidents in the USSR. Take away the political construction of "sluggish schizophrenia" and you take away the disorder. However, there are many other problems which cannot be removed by changing social attitudes, though the problems may come to be seen in relatively more positive or negative lights. For example, in earlier versions of the Diagnostic and Statistical Manual (DSM) homosexuality was seen as a diagnosable mental disorder for which a variety of medical and psychological treatments were offered. However, in recent decades there has been a significant reconstruction of social attitudes to homosexuality in Western cultures such that homosexual disorder is no longer a diagnosis. The "disorder" has therefore disappeared, but that hasn't made homosexuality disappear, only the associated stigma. So, by the same logic, if "schizophrenia" is a socially constructed diagnosis of a stigmatized group, removing the diagnosis and changing the social stigma will not eliminate the problem that some people will hear voices, and a proportion of them will be highly distressed by the experience and will need expert help and support. The modern crusade of the antipsychiatry movement has taken up the issue of schizophrenia as its main battlefield, but each side in the battle has to acknowledge that some people hear voices and that a proportion of such people need expert help. Hearing voices has some similarities with homosexuality, in that certain social constructions, for example in the Middle Ages when hearing voices could be used as evidence of witchcraft, can lead to stigmatization and punishment whereas other social constructions can destigmatize and attract tolerance and support, but there will still be those who need expert support.

So now let's go to the other extreme, the bad biology of the medical model hated by the social constructionists and by some psychologists. The starting question at the level of biology has to be: Are there certain biological mechanisms that can become dysfunctional and thereby impact on psychological and social functioning? Well, the answer to this question is very straightforward, because of course there are such dysfunctional biological mechanisms. These mechanisms are clearly evident in the neurodevelopmental disorders which can have a wide-ranging impact on psychological and social functioning from birth, and in the later acquired neurological disorders in which prior optimal performance at a psychological and social level deteriorates. However, there may be a category difference between neurodevelopmental and acquired neurological disorders and what we have loosely referred to as "madness." If madness, using the majority report approach, includes a construction by an individual and/or by society (either of which can include an "objective" construction that can be generated by a formal diagnostic interview), then in principle a set of organic neurodevelopmental or neurologically acquired disorders should not be labeled as "madness" unless there are some additional problematic features that lead to the construction of "madness" in addition to the basic neurological disorder. For example, let's say that Tom's voices were subsequently discovered to be caused by temporal lobe epilepsy, which had not been diagnosed when he was first labeled as "schizophrenic," but the voices have been cured now that he has been treated with an appropriate anticonvulsant:

> Tom believed himself not to be mad, society (psychiatry) believed him to be mad, but now society (neurology) believes that he is not mad.

In this example, the social construction varies across time from madness to not-madness even though in each case hearing voices was part of Tom's experience. The key point is that a biological sign or symptom in and of itself cannot be used to define "madness," but madness is a subjective or "objective" personal or social construction, which incorporates biological, psychological, or social features. And herein lies the problem for the simple medical model or "objective" approach to madness—that the personal and social constructional aspects of madness mean that it can never in principle be reduced to a set of biological signs, a truth that psychiatry has struggled with for two centuries but still not faced up to.

The starting point for the current approach to madness is therefore that madness is a construction that can include biological, psychological, and social characteristics, but which, in principle, cannot be solely defined at a biomedical level. For example, let's say that we had a monosymptomatic disorder such as a body dysmorphic disorder in which a man believes that his nose is significantly problematic and he wants cosmetic surgery to change it. Although his nose is describable in biomedical terms, there is no inherent biological *sign* that would uniquely identify his nose as problematic, because for any such sign there would be an equivalent nose of similar size, etc., that a different owner would not consider to be dysmorphic. That is, even in such an apparently straightforward case as a body dysmorphic disorder, psychiatry does not deal with biomedical signs but must instead work with *psychological symptoms*. Although many biomedical psychiatrists have, as in Lewis Carroll's story of the hunting of the Snark, spent years searching for the signs of mental illness, their signs have turned out merely to be symptoms, as we will show throughout this book. Psychiatry is therefore a branch of psychology, not a branch of medicine!

Finally, an expression of thanks to all of those psychiatrists and psychologists who over many years have provided challenge and stimulation, though who would no doubt argue strongly against many of the ideas expressed in this book. From my days at the MRC Social Psychiatry Unit I would like to thank John Wing, Paul Bebbington, Robin Murray, Connor Duggan, Julian Leff, and Peter McGuffin, all psychiatrists who have made substantial contributions to our understanding of classification and diagnosis. Subsequently, working in Edinburgh, I have valued many sessions of sparring with Eve Johnstone, David Cunningham Owens, and Chris Freeman. Among my colleagues in psychology I would especially like to thank Tim Dalgleish, Lorna Champion, Andy MacLeod, Charlie Sharp, Ken Laidlaw, Dave Peck, Ann Green, Martin Eisemann, Knut Waterloo, and John Fox. And, finally, my eternal thanks to my children Liam, Jack, and Robyn, to my step-children Anastassiya and Yura, and to my wife Irina who continues to put up with all my strange writing habits.

MICK POWER

CONTENTS

A BRIEF HISTORY OF MADNESS

Love is merely a madness, and I tell you, deserves as well a dark house and whip
as madmen do: and the reason why they are not so punished and cured is, that the
lunacy is so ordinary that the whippers are in love too

Shakespeare, *As You Like It*, Act III, Scene 2, line 386

Introduction

The history of psychiatry is both absurd and grotesque; with the benefit of hindsight, many of its practices have been cruel and inhumane. Nevertheless, each
approach and each treatment was in its time typically based on a proto-scientific
theory that led logically to the practices that were extrapolated from it, such that
we should avoid a "presentist" approach when dealing with the past, with all the
illusions of hindsight that such an approach would appear to offer. For example,
the theory of imbalance of the humors in the blood led naturally to sophisticated
treatises on the appropriate forms of bloodletting for different mental and physical
disorders. Trepanning (the drilling of a hole into the skull) is a practice that archeological evidence reveals has been carried out for thousands of years; it was used to
relieve pressure on the brain, including "mental pressure" (see Figure 1.1). Exorcism
of demons from possessed individuals is also an ancient practice that continues to
the present day. As we will see, in all of these cases expert individuals carried out
the interventions, the interventions were based on theories about human functioning, and even though some people died or were permanently impaired by the
treatments, there were always successful cases that the physician or shaman could
quote to would-be patients and their carers. Such phenomena are examples of what
we would now call *confirmation bias*, in which the patients for whom the treatment
worked are better remembered and more often cited than the ones who died. Doctors bury their mistakes in more ways than one. However, the aim of this chapter on
the history of psychiatry is not simply to present a horror show of cruel treatments
through the ages, but rather to understand each treatment and approach to mental
health in its appropriate historical, cultural, and religious context. Debate about

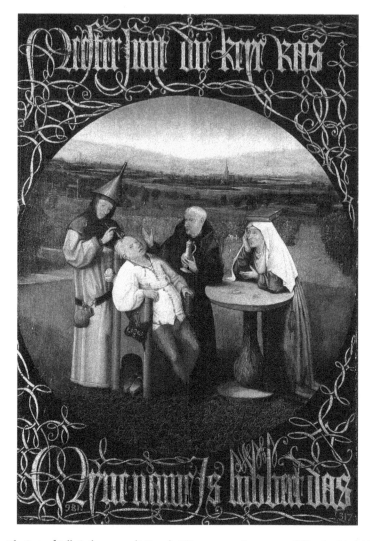

Fig. 1.1. *The Cure of Folly* (oil on panel), Bosch, Hieronymus (*c.*1450–1516)/Prado, Madrid, Spain/
The Bridgeman Art Library.

these different perspectives on mental disorders continues to the present day, so
our remembrance of what is past will help us to master what will be our future.

Early Accounts of Madness

Depression has been known as a disorder for thousands of years. Its earliest known
description comes from the Egyptian wisdom text, *Dispute of a Man With His Ba*, the

papyrus manuscript of which is held in the Berlin State Museum (translation down-loaded from Nederhof, 2009; see also Power, 2012). In this manuscript, a depressed man is arguing with his soul (in ancient Egyptian, the *ba*):

> Look, my soul is disobeying me, while I do not listen to him, is dragging me toward death, before I have come to it, and is throwing me on the fire to burn me up [lines 11–13].

The man then goes on to complain:

> Whom can I talk to today? Faces are blank, every man has his face downcast concern-ing his brothers. Whom can I talk to today? Hearts have become greedy and there is no man's heart on which one may rely [lines 118–121].

Another early vivid description of depression is presented in the Bible when Job loses his possessions and his family, then laments:

> My days are past, my purposes are broken off, even the thoughts of my heart. They change the night into day: the light is short because of darkness. If I wait, the grave is mine house: I have made my bed in the darkness. I have said to corruption, Thou art my father: to the worm, Thou art my mother, and my sister. And where is now my hope? (Job, 17: 11–15)

In the fifth century BCE Hippocrates coined the term "melancholia" (the Latinized form of the original Greek term) to cover this disorder, though he considered it to result from an excess of one of the four humors, black bile, which we will consider shortly. The term "depression" (from the Latin "deprimere" meaning "to press down") was not introduced into English until the seventeenth century. It was popularized by Dr. Johnson in the eighteenth century, but it was only in the late nineteenth and early twentieth centuries in the writings of Griesinger and Kraepelin that the term began to replace "melancholia" as a diagnostic label (see Jackson, 1986, for a detailed history).

Early accounts of what might now be termed schizophrenia can be seen in the Bible and other early texts, though one must apply extreme caution when attempting such a historical diagnosis. In the Book of Daniel we are given the account of Nebuchad-nezzar, the king of Babylon and destroyer of the Temple in Jerusalem. Nebuchadnez-zar has a series of disturbing dreams which none of his own magi are able to interpret, until the captive prophet Daniel provides the necessary insights.

> Nebuchadnezzar dreamed dreams, wherewith his spirit was troubled, and his sleep brake from him (Daniel, 2: 1).

> I saw a dream which made me afraid, and the thoughts upon my bed and the visions of my head troubled me (Daniel, 4: 5).

Daniel tells the king that his dream of a huge statue, with a head of gold, breast and arms of silver, and belly and thighs of brass that breaks into pieces represents the current kingdom of Babylon and then subsequent great kingdoms that will all be destroyed. Nebuchadnezzar's vision of a great tree that is felled is a portent of the king's own fate:

> He was driven from men, and did eat grass as oxen, and his body was wet with the dew of heaven, till his hairs were grown like eagles' feathers, and his nails like birds' claws (Daniel, 4: 33).

The fate that befalls Nebuchadnezzar has been variously interpreted down the centuries, and it speaks volumes about the wishes of the enslaved Jews taken to Babylon and their hope that their god would revenge their defeat by the Babylonians. Nevertheless, the combination of distressing visions, sleep disturbance, and collapse in personal and social functioning provides a dramatic early example of a state that has some similarities to modern-day schizophrenia.

These examples show us that experiences that might now be labeled as depression and schizophrenia have been with us since prehistory, and that the earliest historical references present recognizable descriptions of significant mental distress. In the remainder of this chapter we will begin with early approaches and views of madness that, albeit transformed in certain ways, persist in our diverse views today about the nature of madness.

The Doctrine of the Four Humors

In the pre-Socratic era Empedocles, who lived in the beautiful Greek city of Agrigentum in Sicily, developed the doctrine of the four elements and how the universe is composed of the basic elements of earth, air, fire, and water. According to this idea different combinations of the four elements lead to the great variety of living and non-living structures that we see around us. Empedocles' doctrine of the four elements was the dominant approach for over 2000 years. However, we might note by contrast that the related Chinese view (e.g., Sun-Tzu, 2002) identified five rather than four basic elements of the universe. These were wood, fire, earth, metal, and water; they form the basis of Chinese medicine and Chinese martial arts and are taken into account in the practice of feng shui, which considers the flow of energy between the five elements. The fact that the Greek and Chinese systems have three elements in common suggests that there may have been some exchange of ideas between the different civilizations.

The Greek idea that the universe was composed of four elements was extended to considerations of bodily functioning, initially with the work of Hippocrates

(460–355 BCE), born on the Greek island of Kos, and later extended by Galen (129–200 CE), who was born in Pergamon in present-day Turkey. The doctrine of the four humors, or humorism, considered blood as the equivalent of air, black bile as the equivalent of earth, yellow bile as the equivalent of fire, and phlegm as the equivalent of water. Blood in fact was considered to be composed of all four elements, because if blood is allowed to settle it forms four layers that are derived from the four humors. Applied to psychology, an ideal temperament contained a balanced mixture of the four elements. Galen pointed to four temperaments in which one of the elements predominated, which he named for the humors with which they were associated: the sanguine (an excess of blood), the choleric (an excess of yellow bile), the melancholic (an excess of black bile), and the phlegmatic (an excess of phlegm), terms that are still used today to describe different personalities and that influenced Eysenck's (e.g., Eysenck, 1947) original two-dimensional formulation of personality as stable–neurotic and introvert–extravert. Although the concept of temperament has come to refer primarily to psychological dispositions, the humorists used it to refer to bodily dispositions, which determined a person's susceptibility to particular diseases in addition to their psychological dispositions.

The doctrine of the four humors led to a variety of treatments that followed logically from the theory in attempts to ameliorate a variety of physical and mental ailments. In particular, bloodletting, vomiting, and purging were used from the Hippocratic era onwards until well into the nineteenth century in both Arabic and Christian societies. One approach to bloodletting was to cut a vein close to the supposed diseased part on the same side of the body, such that draining the blood would remove the excess humor. In contrast, the Arabic tradition for bloodletting was to let blood from a vein in the *opposite* side to the supposed diseased part of the body. Interestingly, William Harvey's identification in 1628 of the circulation of the blood, being pumped through the body and brain by the heart, led to an increase in enthusiasm for bloodletting. This included the use of bloodsucking leeches, the method of "cupping" in which cooling air in a cup attached to the skin drew blood to the surface, and even early attempts at blood transfusion which, not surprisingly, usually had a fatal outcome, especially when the transfused blood was obtained from a lamb or a pig (e.g., Jones, 1983). For example, a dominant medieval approach to the treatment of melancholia included the attachment of bloodsucking leeches around the anus. Just the thought of it makes you want to jump up and run, which could have been mistaken for a cure.

Although not strictly part of the doctrine of the four humors, we should also note in this section Plato's comments about the wandering uterus in women and the origins of the concept of "female hysteria" (the word hysteria being derived from the Greek word for uterus). Plato's approach has left its mark on how we view emotion as "irrational" and in conflict with reason, as has been discussed elsewhere (Power and Dalgleish, 2008):

> In men the organ of generation—becoming rebellious and masterful, like an animal dis-obedient to reason, and maddened with the sting of lust—seeks to gain absolute sway; and the same is the case with the . . . womb . . . of women; the animal within them is desirous of procreating children, and when remaining unfruitful long beyond its proper time, gets discontented and angry, and wandering in every direction through the body, closes up the passages of the breath, and by obstructing respiration, drives them to ex-tremity, causing all varieties of diseases (from *The Timaeus*, transl. Jowett, 1953, p. 779).

Again, and in line with the theory, a number of treatments were developed to "cure" the wandering uterus in women so that it returned to its proper place. The famous English herbalist John Gerard (1545–1612) recommended the use of valerian for the treatment of hysteria, because the wandering uterus supposedly disliked the smell of the herb. Plato's link between hysteria and procreation clearly influenced Freud's analyses of the link between the two in his *Studies on Hysteria* published with Josef Breuer in 1895, together with the assumption, since disproved, that hysteria primarily afflicted women.

One important point we should make about the Hippocratic contribution to our understanding of madness is Hippocrates' (and his followers') rejection of madness as divine retribution for sinning against the gods. We will discuss such approaches in the section "Demonic Possession" but, for example, Hippocrates famously questioned the idea that epilepsy was of divine origin, the so-called sacred disease, but instead had natural causes:

> It is thus with regard divine no more sacred than other diseases, but has a natural cause from the originates like other affections. Men regard its nature and cause as divine from ignorance and wonder (Hippocrates, *On the Sacred Disease*).

Again, it is understandable that a seizure attack could be construed as some form of demonic possession, or that the visions that can accompany some forms of epilepsy could be interpreted as sent by the gods. Indeed, religious visionaries such as St. Paul, St. Teresa of Avila, and Muhammad have been assumed by many to have suffered from epilepsy (Power, 2012).

Demonic Possession

The idea that all forms of illness may be the result of supernatural intervention reaches back to our earliest prehistory, with the discovery, for example, of the early use of trepanning possibly being used to allow demons to escape from the brain. Homer (*c.*1000 BCE) considered that people suffering from insanity had offended the gods who then punished them by making them behave strangely. Even today our innocent statement of "bless you!" (originally "God bless you!") when someone sneezes acknowledges this ancient tradition with the belief that the sneeze is a result of demons escaping from the body. Ancient cave paintings in places such as Altamira and Lascaux portray people wearing animal head-dresses, which have been interpreted (e.g., Lewis-Williams, 2010) to represent priest-shamans who attempted to bring good fortune to those involved in the dangers of the hunt. The priest-shaman role continues in many traditional societies, with beliefs in supernatural possession often existing alongside the use of modern medicine, and these may offer some insight into more ancient practices.

The shaman and the patient share a world view in which, for example, evil spirits are believed to have entered the patient and their removal depends on the skill and experience of the shaman. Jerome Frank presents a detailed analysis of the treatment of "espanto" (similar to agitated depression) in a Guatemalan Indian woman (Frank, 1973, pp. 59–62). The treatment took the form of a group healing ceremony that was attended not just by the patient but also, as Frank notes, by her husband, a male friend, and two anthropologists. At the initial meeting the shaman made the diagnosis of "espanto." The group ceremony took place in the patient's house and lasted over 12 hours until late into the night. The shaman made wax dolls of the evil spirits, then massaged the patient with eggs, which were believed to absorb the sickness from the patient's body. At 2 a.m. the patient was taken outside semi-naked and sprayed with a "magic fluid" that had a high alcohol content, so that she quickly became very cold. She also drank a pint of the magic fluid. She was taken back into her house, where she was massaged again with the eggs in order to absorb the remaining sickness. The shaman then broke the eggs into water one-by-one, declaring that the espanto would be cured as the eggs fell to the bottom of the bowl. As it turned out, the next day the patient developed a high fever, which the anthropologists treated with antibiotics, but within a few days she had recovered from both the fever and the espanto or depression.

Within Christianity, the ritual of exorcism bears many similarities to some of the traditional healing ceremonies in which evil spirits or demons are removed from the sufferer's body. The Christian tradition of exorcism begins in the Bible with Jesus famously casting out demons on several occasions, as in the case of the Gadarene swine when he cast devils out of a man from Gadarene into a herd of swine who then ran into the Sea of Galilee and drowned themselves:

> And they came over unto the other side of the sea, into the country of the Gadarenes … immediately there met him out of the tombs a man with an unclean spirit … He said unto him, Come out of the man thou unclean spirit. And he asked him, What is thy name? And he answered, saying, My name is Legion: for we are many … And forthwith

Jesus gave them leave. And the unclean spirits went out, and entered into the swine; and the herd ran violently down a steep place into the sea, (they were about two thousand;) and were choked in the sea (Mark, 5: 1–13).

By the third century CE a special group of clerics, known as exorcists, had emerged in the Christian Church. Their function was to cast out evil spirits from the afflicted. At that time the ceremony of baptism included a ritual for exorcism, because original sin, which Christianity teaches every person is born with, was believed in part to result from the influence of the devil. Ritual exorcism is still used in today's Christian churches to differing degrees; for example, a version of exorcism, the deliverance ceremony, is commonly used in the Charismatic Christian movement to help individuals overcome evil influences, a practice that became more common after the film *The Exorcist* was released in 1973. In Catholicism, the Roman Ritual is spelt out in the book *Of Exorcisms and Certain Supplications*, which was revised as recently as 1998 having been left untouched since 1614. Exorcism is also carried out in other religions, including Hinduism, some forms of Buddhism, Islam, and Judaism. The take-home message from studies of shamanism, exorcism, psychotherapy, and the placebo effect in medicine is that people's world beliefs have a major impact on their understanding of health and illness (Frank, 1973). Therefore, curative rituals which are consistent with those world views may have a positive health-enhancing and spiritually uplifting effect for those people when they have engaged in ritual practices led by a shaman, a priest, a psychotherapist, or medical doctor. Jerome Frank made these links explicit in *Persuasion and Healing* in a way that helps us to understand why religious healing practices can clearly benefit some of the people who seek help, though it is likely that the mechanisms of such benefit include the placebo effect and other effects that belief can engender.

The pursuit of witches, especially in the Middle Ages, was fuelled by the belief that these women were possessed by the devil and therefore needed to be "cured" of the madness of witchcraft. There are of course many other examples of misogyny throughout the world's religions but the institutionalized misogyny that is part of the Christian Church clearly reached its peak in the Middle Ages. The publication in 1487 of the *Malleus Maleficarum* (*The Hammer of Witches*) by two Dominican monks, Heinrich Kramer and Jacob Sprenger, provided a handbook for the detection, interrogation, and torture of witches. The Dominican order had been assigned as the inquisitors by Pope Gregory IX in the thirteenth century, a task at which they excelled, to the extent that they were known at that time as the "Domini canes," which translates as the "hounds of the Lord." Estimates of the number of women accused of witchcraft who were put to death in the sixteenth and seventeenth centuries range from 50,000 to 200,000. Infamous witch trials such as those in Salem, Massachusetts, are remembered to this day. In 1590, North Berwick near Edinburgh, Scotland, today a pleasant seaside town, witnessed witch trials in which over 100 people were accused of witchcraft, all because while travelling back from Denmark King James VI had experienced bad storms at sea which were blamed on witches in North Berwick. The North Berwick trials were the first major witchcraft trials in Scotland, and although there were some men included among the accused by far the majority were women. One such woman was Agnes Sampson who was brought to the palace of King James at Holyrood House in Edinburgh where she was held in a witch's bridle, with a rope around her neck, and prevented from sleeping. Following successful torture, Agnes subsequently confessed to 53 crimes of witchcraft, despite having worked as a respected healer and midwife in her community. On January 16, 1590, she was hung, garroted, and then burnt to ashes.

Another example of a psychological phenomenon that has been interpreted as demonic possession, similar to the earlier accounts of epilepsy, is that of the fugue state (see Power, 2012). A fugue state is a rare phenomenon in which a person suffers an amnesic episode and usually travels away from home and can assume a new identity. The state normally lasts a matter of hours or days, but in some cases has been documented to last for years. There is normally an abrupt return of the previous self with an amnesia for the time spent in the fugue state. The fugue state is normally precipitated by a personal crisis or stress and is not related to substance abuse or other medical conditions because it is of psychological origin. The writer Agatha Christie is believed to have suffered such a fugue when she disappeared from her home in Cornwall and then appeared in Harrogate in Yorkshire 12 days later but with no memory for the intervening period.

It seems likely that the fugue state has been one of the sources of so-called mystical states, especially in which the person has become "possessed" by another identity (though we note that there are many other types of and possible sources of mystical states; see Power, 2012). Fugue states and trance states have been well documented in the anthropological literature in religious and shamanic practices. The anthropologist Michael Lambek in *Human Spirits: A Cultural Account of Trance in Mayotte* (Lambek, 1981) describes trance behavior among the inhabitants of Mayotte, a small island in the Comoro Archipelago in the Indian Ocean. Lambek describes how the people of Mayotte (usually the women in the group) enter into trance states, during which they believe their bodies are inhabited by spirits. The trance can best be understood as a social activity within a defined system of cultural meaning rather than as a "psychological problem." However, his descriptions of "trance" include the absence of the person who becomes incommunicado and who a spirit has taken over as a new identity. The Mayotte spirits will then talk to the villagers and hold conversations with them, but the entranced person has no recollection of the spirit or the conversation afterwards.

One way that those who participate in Haitian voodoo may enter a fugue state is to become possessed by the loa, one of the religion's spirits. When the loa possesses someone, their body is considered as being used by the spirit. These spirits can offer prophecies of future events and situations. Practitioners experience such possession to be an exhausting experience. The possessed person has no recollection of the possession and normally suffers amnesia for the time of the possession. It is said that only the spirit can choose who it wants to possess and that those who become possessed have a high spiritual level. The voodoo notion of the zombie, which has proven so popular among Hollywood film-makers, also presents many features of the fugue state. The zombie is considered to be a corpse that has been raised from the dead and that, at least in Haiti, seems to have been used to carry out some of the more boring and tiring agricultural work that the African slaves were originally brought to the Caribbean and Americas to do. It is also believed that there are those who feign possession because they want attention and status, therefore a "chwal" will undergo some form of trial or testing to make sure that the possession is indeed genuine. For example, someone who claims to be possessed by one of the spirits may be offered a liqueur made by steeping chili peppers in alcohol. If the possessed person consumes the liqueur without showing any evidence of pain or discomfort, the possession is considered to be genuine. The most important voodoo ceremony in Haitian history was in August 1791 and began the Haitian Revolution. In this ceremony a spirit loa possessed a priestess and received a pig sacrificed as an offering. All who were present at the ceremony pledged themselves to fight for the freedom of the slaves and against French colonial rule; this was eventually achieved in 1804 with the establishment of the Republic of Haiti, the first black people's republic formed as the result of a successful slave revolt.

Finally, we should note that during their lifetimes many of the now-venerated Christian mystics were often accused of witchcraft or demonic possession. For example, consider the case of Margery Kempe (*c*.1373–*c*.1440) who dictated the events of her life as she neared death because she could neither read nor write and in doing so produced not only the first autobiography in the English language but also one of the most extraordinary autobiographies that has ever been written. The manuscript of *The Book of Margery Kempe* (Kempe, 2004) lay forgotten for hundreds of years and was only rediscovered in 1934 by an American medieval scholar, Hope Emily Allen, in the private library of the Butler-Bowdons in Lancashire. The autobiography begins with Kempe's account of her breakdown shortly after the birth of the first of her 14 children, in what is now King's Lynn in Norfolk. During this breakdown she began to hallucinate, seeing devils around her, and had to be chained up for 6 months because of fears for her own safety. This postpuerperal condition seems to have been resolved when Christ appeared to her and talked to her, persuading her to return to him. After further years of ambivalence about her calling, with accounts of a failed brewery and a series of sexual temptations, she eventually negotiated a life of celibacy with her husband and then proceeded to travel around all of the main pilgrimage sites in Europe and the Holy Land. She recorded her visits to other notable mystics of the time, including Julian of Norwich. However, during all of these travels and visits, Kempe has numerous conversations with Christ, which are recorded in her book, as well as seeming to alienate most people she ever travelled with because of her constant weeping and wailing, which she could break into at disconcerting times:

> She had so much feeling for the manhood of Christ, that when she saw women in Rome carrying children in their arms, if she could discover that any were boys, she would cry, roar and weep as if she had seen Christ in his childhood. And if she could have had her way, she would often have taken the children out of their mothers' arms and kissed them instead of Christ ... And therefore she cried many times and often when she met a handsome man, and wept and sobbed bitterly for the manhood of Christ as she went about the streets of Rome, so that those who saw her were greatly astonished at her, because they did not know the reason (Kempe, 2004, p. 123).

The sexual nature of her relationship with Christ is similar to that found with other Christian female mystics such as St. Teresa of Avila (Power, 2012); for example, Kempe reports Christ saying the following to her:

> Therefore I must be intimate with you, and lie in your bed with you. Daughter, you greatly desire to see me, and you may boldly, when you are in bed, take me to you as your wedded husband, as your dear darling ... and I want you to love me, daughter, as a good wife ought to love her husband. Therefore you can boldly take me in the arms of your soul and kiss my mouth, my head, and my feet as sweetly as you want (Kempe, 2004, p. 127).

By modern-day standards Margery would of course meet a number of possible psychiatric diagnostic criteria, including schizophrenia, puerperal psychosis, and schizo-affective psychosis. In medieval Europe she divided opinion equally between those who saw her as mystic saint and those who saw her as demonically possessed; thus, she underwent religious interrogation on several occasions, was imprisoned, and nearly burnt at the stake several times for heresy, only to be saved by the efforts of her supporters who protected her.

"Holistic" Treatments in Sacred Caves and Temples

The method of "incubation" was used in ancient Egypt and Greece and typically consisted of sleep, the "balm of hurt minds" as Shakespeare referred to it in Macbeth, and dream interpretation by priest-physicians (e.g., Ellenberger, 1970). The afflicted person would spend the night in a sacred cave or temple such as in the Greek temples of Asclepios in Epidaurus and Pergamon. Various rituals, included statues that appeared to move, sounds, and the burning of herbs and incense, were all used to provoke rich dreams for interpretation in the morning. A famous example quoted in the Bible is when Solomon visited the temple in Gibeon, a city just north of Jerusalem:

> And the king went to Gibeon to sacrifice there; for that was the great high place: a thousand burnt offerings did Solomon offer upon that altar. In Gibeon the Lord appeared to Solomon in a dream by night: and God said, Ask what I shall give thee. And Solomon said . . . Give therefore thy servant an understanding heart to judge thy people, that I may discern between good and bad (Kings, 3: 4–9).

After which account follows the famous story of Solomon and the two women arguing over a baby, which he threatens to cut in two and give half to each.

There are many healing traditions that have developed from these Greek and Egyptian traditions which include the notion of special places of healing. In fact the use of natural springs and caves as sacred places of healing may have had some rationale behind them because of the special mineral content in many of the sacred springs that were developed as spas. For example, during their occupation of England the Romans developed the site of an ancient Celtic spring dedicated to the goddess Sulis into the Roman town of Bath, which was then devoted to the syncretic goddess Sulis-Minerva. The Roman baths are still a popular visitor attraction, with the hot and somewhat sulfurous water that emerges from the spring providing an interesting medicinal challenge for those who wish to drink it.

The links between the sacred and the healing have continued throughout history, with places of religious pilgrimage, holy relics, and the development of churches and monasteries in often dramatic locations adding to belief in their healing powers (e.g., Power, 2012). For example, the monastic movement that developed in religions such as Christianity initially saw the rise of the desert hermits, like St. Antony among the Coptic Christians in Egypt. The movement developed with later leaders such as St. Basil of Caesarea, who devised the coenobitical community rules that reached their pinnacle with the Rule of St. Benedict (480–550 CE)—Benedict being an Italian monk whose hagiography by Pope Gregory the Great led to his cult status and the development of the Benedictine movement. The monasteries that arose out of this movement were typically places of learning. The Grande Chartreuse is the leading monastery of the Carthusian movement founded by St. Bruno in the eleventh century and located in a beautiful but remote mountain valley in the Isere region in the south of France. To quote Guigo of Grenoble, one of its early priors, "books are . . . the everlasting food of our souls. We wish them to be most carefully kept and to be zealously made" (quoted in Lawrence, 2001, p. 159). As well as books, the Carthusians of Chartreuse also gave us the wonderful green Chartreuse liqueur made from distilled alcohol and about 130 different herb and floral extracts, which although originally intended as a medicine has been put to a variety of non-medicinal uses since. Most of the monasteries would have a herb garden and a dispensary for helping the sick, some even offering an infirmary.

The Priory of St. Mary of Bethlehem was a monastery founded in 1247 in Bishopsgate London, though it has moved several times in its history, its current location being Beckenham in southeast London. From 1330 it functioned as a hospital such that it is now one of the world's oldest psychiatric institutions. Under its infamous name "Bedlam," the Bethlem Hospital became synonymous with the worst excesses of madness and the mistreatment of the insane across the centuries. Until the eighteenth century, Bethlem was the only psychiatric hospital in Britain, but then provision began to be made by other hospitals such as Thomas Guy's, which, when founded in London in 1728, included provision for "20 lunatic incurables." Hospitals such as the Bethlem in London and the Bicêtre in Paris became fashionable forms of entertainment during this period, with the Bicêtre attracting as many as 2000 paying guests on a Sunday. However, there was little in the way of treatment, with the chief physician attending maybe once a year, for example, to prescribe bloodletting in the spring or purging in the autumn (Jones, 1983). We will return later in the chapter, in the section "The Asylum Movement," to consider the rise of asylums from the eighteenth century onwards.

"Shock" Treatments

The recognition of the circulation of the blood by William Harvey in 1628 led to similar proposals for the operation of a separate system of nerves, which were beginning to be understood for their role in the control of action and the detection of stimulation. Phrases still in use today, such as "What he needs is a good shake," originate from this viewpoint. For example, Rene Descartes (e.g., Descartes, 1649) believed that the nerves were very fine tubes along which nerve fluids ran to provide mechanical control of the body. In his description of the example of fear, in which we run and feel frightened, he suggests:

> Simply in virtue of the fact that certain spirits proceed at the same time toward the nerves that move the legs to flee, they cause another movement in the same gland by means of which the soul feels and perceives this flight—which can in this way be excited in the body merely by the disposition of the organs (Descartes, 1649, Article 38).

As with other theories that we have considered, such as the imbalance of the four humors leading to the use of bloodletting as a treatment, the proposal that nervous problems could arise from the nerve fluid being trapped or caught in the tiny pipes that constituted the nervous system led to obvious forms of treatment that were designed to "shock" the fluid into movement.

One of the earlier approaches to shock treatment was noted above, when we considered the use of foul-smelling herbs such as valerian to shock the wandering uterus back into its proper place in the treatment of hysteria. Sudden plunging into cold water was one form of treatment, but the approach taken was that the more surprising the plunge then the more effective the treatment; thus, elaborate mechanisms were designed that included bridges over cold ponds or rivers that collapsed unexpectedly, thereby hurtling the patient into the water. Boats were built in which groups of patients were floated out into lakes, but then the boats broke up throwing their occupants into the water. In 1880 such hydrotherapy was still in use in Killarney in Ireland, when a manic women was tied behind a boat and towed across a freezing lake, but unfortunately she developed pneumonia and died from the treatment. Rotatory machines, such as the one shown in Figure 1.2, were designed on the assumption that fast and lengthy rotation would eventually force the trapped fluids in the nerves to move. Erasmus Darwin (1731–1802) suggested that for congestion of the brain the head should be outermost in rotation, whereas for congestion of the internal organs the feet should be outwards.

Another favorite form of "shock" treatment consisted of beatings and floggings, again on the assumption that nervous fluid trapped in certain parts of the body would

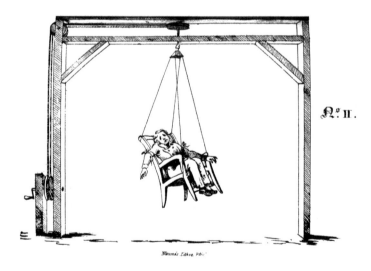

Fig. 1.2. The Rotatory Machine from Alexander Morison, *Cases of Mental Disease*, 1828. © The British Library Board.

become unstuck. Paying visitors to the Bethlem Hospital were often entertained with such treatment of the inmates. Electrical shock treatment seems to have been known since Galen reportedly used an electric fish to treat melancholy (Jackson, 1986). Electrical machines that produced static electricity became fashionable in medicine in the eighteenth century, with the Electrical Dispensary, founded in London in 1793, becoming big business. A surgeon at St. Thomas's Hospital in London, John Birch, reported the cure of two melancholics using such electrical treatment. Benjamin Franklin (1706–90), who famously conducted experiments involving flying kites during thunderstorms to show their true nature, knocked himself out on several occasions during his experiments and is reported to have recommended "trying the practice on mad people." Although the development of electroconvulsive therapy (ECT) by Ugo Cerletti in the twentieth century may not have been based on Descartes' trapped fluid proposal (indeed ECT does not seem to be based on any theory whatsoever), it does continue in the tradition of administering painful and unacceptably large shocks to vulnerable patients. The mistaken idea that sufferers from epilepsy did not experience schizophrenia seems to have suggested to Cerletti and others that the artificial creation of seizures through electrical currents would therefore be a treatment for schizophrenia, which does have a twisted logic, not least because people with epilepsy can experience schizophrenia. However, any form of "shock" treatment should not be dismissed as simply barbaric or ineffective: first because the various forms of shock treatment followed logically from the theory of trapped nervous fluid, and second because treatments such as ECT have been shown, for example in the work of Eve Johnstone and colleagues (Johnstone et al., 1980), to be effective in some cases of severe depression.

The Asylum Movement

We have already noted that at the beginning of the eighteenth century there was only one psychiatric hospital in Britain, the Bethlem. However, by the end of the century there were 15 such hospitals, as the so-called great confinement began, as put forward Michel Foucault in his book *Madness and Civilization* (Foucault, 1971). Foucault's controversial analysis proposed that societies need stigmatized groups. The stigmatized group in earlier centuries had been lepers who had been confined in lazar houses or sent to leper colonies, but in Britain the dissolution of the monasteries under Henry VIII had been accompanied by the loss of the lazar houses with a subsequent shift toward stigmatization of the mad and the poor instead. Foucault's analysis has been widely debated and criticized, but perhaps the most important point is that as a constructionist Foucault deliberately reconstructs the past, so perhaps we should leave the constructionists to be hoist by their own petards. Nevertheless, Foucault provides an important perspective on our treatment of madness as the Age of Reason began and continues to the present day.

In Britain, most of the psychiatric hospitals that developed in the eighteenth century were private establishments that varied considerably in their conditions and treatment according to the wealth or poverty of the inmates and their families. Only through an Act of Parliament in 1808 were public funds allocated for the development of asylums with a further Act in 1845 making it mandatory for each county to have asylum provision (e.g., Porter, 2002). Many such asylums were opened with well-intentioned principles. For example, the Middlesex County Asylum, known as the Hanwell Pauper and Lunatic Asylum, opened in 1831 for a group of 300 patients. Its first superintendent, William Ellis, believed that fresh air and exercise were important for recovery from madness, so the hospital grounds were developed with pleasant gardens and walkways. He also believed that "therapeutic employment" was also part of the recovery and the hospital became a near self-sufficient community which included agriculture, a bakery, and a brewery in which the inmates worked as part of their rehabilitation. Its next superintendent, John Connolly, became well known for his removal of the use of restraints for inmates, which was a widespread practice in asylums up until that time. Connolly was undoubtedly influenced by the great French psychiatrist Philippe Pinel (1745–1826) who was appalled by the conditions and use of restraint at the Bicêtre psychiatric hospital in Paris, where for example he found one patient who had been in chains for 40 years.

Another such famous and well-intentioned asylum was opened by the Quaker Tuke family in York in 1792. The founder, William Tuke, was a tea merchant who wanted to re-create, as Porter (2002) has noted, an ideal bourgeois family home for patients and staff, who all lived, worked, and dined together. The York Retreat was initially available only for Quakers, but later on opened its doors to non-Quakers too. The approach taken used minimal restraint and minimal medical intervention. As Samuel Tuke, William' Tuke's grandson stated: "The physician plainly perceived how much was to be done by moral and how little by medical means" (quoted in Porter, 1990, p. 223). There are many hagiographies of the York Retreat and the whole Moral Therapy or Moral Management movement, as it came to be called, but it is also important to consider the subsequent Victorian extremes to which this movement went. The patients at the York Retreat were treated like children who were to be re-socialized into good Quaker ways. Learning self-restraint by internalizing the external discipline was a primary goal of treatment. As Foucault stated, moral therapy replaced the manacles of iron with manacles of the mind, the "mind-forg'd manacles" that formed the title of Roy Porter's (1990) classic book. A new form of insanity "moral insanity" becomes a type of diagnosis, with associated types such as "masturbational insanity," or Onanism from Onan in the Book of Genesis who "spilled his seed" rather than impregnating his brother's wife, reflecting the challenge that sexuality posed for the Victorian age. To quote from Henry Maudsley, founder of the Maudsley Hospital:

> the development of puberty may indirectly lead to insanity by becoming the occasion of a vicious habit of self-abuse (Maudsley, 1870, pp. 86–87).

Since the eighteenth century masturbation had been thought to cause physical weakness and even a risk of blindness, but the Victorian age took it into a form of insanity for which moral exhortation and the teaching of self-restraint formed the initial Moral Management approach. Nymphomania was an equivalent diagnosis in women, who would be physically examined to see if they had enlarged clitorises, in which case a clitoridectomy was often performed (see for example *The Madness of Women* by Jane Ussher, 2011). Treatment of masturbation in men included shock treatment, the use of restraining devices, and even removal of the genitals if other measures did not work. Circumcision became widely used in the USA and UK during Victorian times because it was considered to reduce the likelihood of masturbation.

The nineteenth century witnessed a massive expansion in the size and number of asylums. The Hanwell Asylum that was mentioned earlier was opened in 1831 for approximately 300 patients, but by the end of the nineteenth century it had expanded to cater for over 2000 patients. These increases continued well into the twentieth century. When Erving Goffman was carrying out research for his famous book *Asylums* (Goffman, 1961), he did a year's field work from 1955–6 at St. Elizabeth's Hospital in Washington D.C., which at that stage had more than 7000 inmates. The inmates of these huge institutions continued from the nineteenth century onwards to consist of a wide range of cases that would no longer be considered psychiatric disorders. For example, Mary Boyle in her *Schizophrenia: A Scientific Delusion* (Boyle, 2002) argued (though not without dispute; see, for example, Turner, 2003) that many of the so-called schizophrenics studied by the greats of psychiatry such as Kraepelin and Bleuler first of all included a substantial number of cases of tertiary syphilis, known then as general paresis of the insane but finally recognized by Noguchi in 1913 to be a consequence of the syphilis spirochete. Secondly, these "schizophrenic" patients included large numbers of people infected in epidemics of the viral disease encephalitis lethargica. There were various waves of this infection in the nineteenth and twentieth centuries, with estimates suggesting that more people died from this viral infection in the great epidemic just after the First World War than died in the First World War itself. Some might argue that it was no fault of psychiatry at that time that infectious causes of psychiatric-like symptoms were not understood, even though these days patients would more likely be treated by neurologists rather than psychiatrists.

The present day has seen the closure of most of the asylums worldwide. They have been replaced by a variety of systems of "community care" that include relatively short-stay psychiatric units and hospitals for acute psychiatric treatment, out-patient and day-patient units, and hostels often based in the poorest and most deprived parts of the community. There were a number of both positive and negative factors that led to the decline and closure of the large asylums from the 1950s onwards. Psychiatry would point to the development of psychotropic medication such as chlorpromazine in the 1950s, as we will discuss in more detail in the next section "Pharmacotherapy," although skeptics would say that this was more coincidence than cause (e.g., Boyle, 2002). The clear recognition in the classic works by people like Erving Goffman, John Wing, and George Brown of the consequences of institutionalization contributed substantially to the community care movement. However, the downside was that the large asylums were extremely expensive and draining on healthcare resources, such that prime city sites were often closed and sold off at considerable profit without any obvious benefit or development of replacement community services.

Pharmacotherapy

All societies at all times seem to have discovered the delights of alcohol from the natural fermentation of the sugars in fruit, and from the fermentation of grains. Breakfast for the average Egyptian pyramid builder is estimated to have included the equivalent of two pints of beer produced in the local village brewery (e.g., Wilkinson, 2010). And when the Arabic alchemist Gabir Ibn Hayan (702–65 CE) distilled fermented grape juice and declared that he had finally discovered the "elixir of life," he had of course discovered how to make a good brandy with a method of distillation that soon became popular in other cultures too. These distillates, or early forms of brandy, gin, whisky, schnapps, vodka, and grappa, provided the basis for many pharmacological treatments for many centuries, the famous Chartreuse from the Cluniac monastery in the south of France that was mentioned earlier being one such example. A similar product, originally produced by the Benedictine monks of Buckfast Abbey in Devon and called Buckfast Tonic Wine is used as a "medication," especially at the weekends, by many teenagers even today. It is known in Scotland under a variety of names including "wreck the hoose juice," "commotion lotion," and "Coatbridge table wine."

Until the nineteenth century, in addition to alcohol, most pharmacological treatments consisted of a variety of herbal remedies. Theophrastus (c.300 BCE) presented a list of 500 plants with curative properties that formed the basis for subsequent and present-day herbal remedies. For example, the Greeks made use of hellebore, an extract from the Christmas rose which causes violent purging and vomiting, in order to cleanse the body. Pliny the Elder (23–79 CE) expanded Theophrastus' list to 1000 plants. An extract of one species of the poppy plant, opium, has been popular since ancient times for its sedative and hypnotic qualities. A mixture of opium and alcohol known as laudanum was very popular as a Victorian nightcap and was used in some of the asylums. The nineteenth century also witnessed considerable developments in chemistry, with morphine being isolated in 1803, chloral hydrate synthesized by Von Liebig in 1832, and phenothiazine synthesized in 1883. The phenothiazines were initially developed as artificial dyes, but scientists at the firm Du Pont discovered that they had insecticidal properties and phenothiazine was introduced as an insecticide in 1935. The phenothiazine chlorpromazine was first synthesized in 1950, and was one in a sequence of phenothiazines that the French company Laboratoires Rhone-Poulenc were developing as antihistamines. The French surgeon Henri Laborit tested chlorpromazine as an anesthetic booster in a military hospital in Paris. He noted its subsequent calming effect on his patients, so then began testing it with a variety of other disorders including psychiatric disorders. Jean Delay and Pierre Deniker at the neighboring Sainte-Anne hospital heard about Laborit's work and tested the drug on 38 patients with manic and acute psychotic states. They published their dramatic results in 1952, following which Delay and Laborit seem to have spent the rest of their lives in dispute about who made the clinical discovery. As David Healy (2008) notes, this dispute probably cost them any share of a Nobel Prize that might otherwise have been awarded.

A second line of development of the colorful insecticidal phenothiazines occurred when the Swiss company Geigy produced a new phenothiazine called imipramine. Although it seemed ineffective with agitated psychotic states—indeed it even seemed to make some patients more agitated—possible benefits for the treatment of depression were noted. The Swiss psychiatrist Roland Kuhn tested the chemical with hospitalized melancholic patients, and published positive findings in 1957. The tricyclic benzene rings within the chemical structure led to imipramine being the first of a series of related tricyclic antidepressants that subsequently included other tricyclics such as amitriptyline, clomipramine, and nortriptyline.

The scale of the modern pharmaceutical industry has no comparison, other than with the current drug, alcohol, and tobacco industries. Figures on industry revenues (see, for example, <http://www.vfa.de/en/statistics/>) show that over US$640 billion were spent globally on prescription drugs in 2006. Almost half of this market is accounted for by the USA which spent nearly US$290 billion; this represented a continuing increase in profits, and with other industries going into financial downturn the pharmaceutical industries are among the most profitable in the USA. The major drugs sold worldwide include Pfizer's anticholesterol drug Lipitor with global sales of nearly US$13 billion, followed by Plavix, an anticoagulant from Bristol Myers Squibb, and Nexium, and antiheartburn pill from AstraZeneca. In terms of total revenue, Pfizer leads the pack with nearly US$68 billion in 2006, followed by Novartis with US$53 billion, Merck and Co. at US$46 billion, and Bayer at US$44 billion. To put these figures in context, the estimated gross domestic product for Mali, one of the world's poorest countries, was estimated at US$14.8 billion in 2006. Our pursuit of health and happiness is very big business indeed and it exists on a scale that puts many of the world's poorest countries into the shade.

It would be possible to examine the evidence for each of the pharmaceutical industry's major drugs and ask to what extent it has improved the world's mental health and happiness. For example, on the basis of the record consumption of prescription medicines in the USA, if the equations were that simple then the USA should have the most long-lived and happiest population of any nation by a long way. In fact, the opposite is the case, as shown in the work summarized by Wilkinson and Pickett (2010). The longevity figures alone show that the USA trails some way behind most of Europe and Japan, so their heavy consumption of pharmaceuticals is not having the desired effect. However, rather than examine all prescription medicines with all their exaggerated claims and flaws, we will focus on mental health pharmaceuticals because they are explicitly marketed for the replacement of misery with happiness (see Power, in press). And no pharmaceutical in this realm has gained as much notoriety as Prozac, so we will now briefly consider the Prozac story.

The story of Prozac began in the Eli Lilly laboratories in the early 1970s when it was recognized that one of their antihistamines, diphenhydramine, as in the earlier phenothiazine work, seemed to show some antidepressant properties. One of the Eli Lilly scientists, David Wong, developed a substance intended to inhibit uptake of the neurotransmitter serotonin, and published the first article on the newly named fluoxetine in 1974; this was given the trade name Prozac in 1975. The drug was eventually approved by the United States Food and Drug Administration (US FDA) in 1987, following which Eli Lilly began selling it, with sales in the USA reaching US$350 million within a year. However, Eli Lilly's claim that they had developed the first selective serotonin reuptake inhibitor (SSRI) had to be corrected because an earlier SSRI, zimelidine, had been produced previously.

However, the controversy that has surrounded Prozac has not been limited to whether or not it was the first SSRI, but has included a range of critical clinical issues, some of which have not been fully resolved. The first of these relates to the evidence base for the use of Prozac for depression in adults. Current UK National Institute for

Health and Care Excellence (NICE) guidelines only recommend pharmacological treatments such as Prozac as first-line treatments for severe depression (National Institute for Health and Care Excellence, 2009). This recommendation is supported by a recent meta-analysis, which did not demonstrate the efficacy of antidepressants in minor to moderate depression (Barbui et al., 2011). However, the recommendations also state that treatment should be continued for 6 months following remission of symptoms. Continuing treatment with antidepressants reduces the odds of relapse by 70% compared with treatment discontinuation (Geddes et al., 2003). Choosing among the different available antidepressants has not previously been evidence based, but a meta-analysis in 2009 offered some guidance. Cipriani et al. (2009) investigated the acute treatment of unipolar major depression with 12 new-generation antidepressants. Mirtazapine, escitalopram, venlafaxine, and sertraline were found to be significantly more efficacious than Prozac and a number of other antidepressants. Escitalopram and sertraline were the best accepted and hence less discontinued than antidepressants such as Prozac because of side effects from the medication. In general, the choice of antidepressant depends on issues such as previous beneficial response, side effects, and tolerability. A randomized placebo-controlled trial of cognitive behavioral therapy (CBT) and Prozac found that pharmacotherapy alone reduced depression by only 18–21% compared with placebo but that combined treatment did not reduce the risk of relapse of moderate depressive disorder, which again points to the use of antidepressants such as Prozac only in severe cases of depression (Petersen et al., 2004).

The second clinical controversy surrounding Prozac is whether or not it increases the risk of suicide and homicide in adults. A famous case in 1989 led to a protracted law suit against Eli Lilly that was not settled until 1994. The case involved Joseph Wesbecker in Louisville Kentucky, who had been taking Prozac for 4 weeks when he went to his place of work, a printing company named Standard Gravure, and with a semi-automatic rifle and a number of pistols opened fire on the staff working in the plant. Not long before, Standard Gravure had been in the news because it had been bought out by Michael Shea; he had used US$11 million from the employees' pension fund to enable the purchase of the printing works. During a 30-minute shooting spree Wesbecker killed 7 and injured 12 of the workers in the plant and then shot himself. As part of the legal proceedings against Eli Lilly and Prozac, Eli Lilly were forced to release internal company documents that had begun to chart the risks of suicide, homicide, and increased violence linked with Prozac; these documents were then used as evidence in further legal cases against Eli Lilly. The Prozac Survivors Group documented hundreds of such cases in the 1990s—people who had suffered from increased violence against self and others, increased suicidal ideation, and increased suicide attempts. More recent summaries of the evidence suggest that, in adults, the net effect seems to be neutral on suicidal behavior but possibly protective for suicidal ideation (Gibbons et al., 2012; Stone et al., 2009). In a large Finnish cohort study, Tiihonen et al. (2006) found a substantially lower mortality during SSRI use, but among subjects who had ever used an antidepressant there was an increased risk of attempted suicide (39%) even if completed suicide was reduced.

The third clinical controversy has been about the use of Prozac in children and adolescents. The risk of suicidality associated with use of antidepressants appears to be strongly age dependent, with adolescents at particular risk. In the early 2000s claims that SSRIs increased suicidal behavior threatened their reputation as "safer" antidepressants. The US FDA issued a so-called black box warning for antidepressants in relation to the risk of suicidal thoughts and behavior in children and young adults following these concerns. Paroxetine and fluoxetine were particularly implicated, with their short half-lives and significant withdrawal symptoms, which can be problematic where there is some erratic use of the medication in which the child or adolescent can be regularly going into a state of withdrawal. In children aged 10–19 years there was also a reported increased risk of death with paroxetine use (with an increased risk ratio of over 5.4). The UK NICE guidelines for treatment of depression in children and young people (National Institute for Health and Care Excellence, 2005) state that antidepressant medication should not be used for the initial treatment of children and adolescents with mild depression, and that if they have moderate to severe depression that the treatment offered should be a psychological therapy such as CBT, interpersonal psychotherapy, or family therapy.

This level of detail is necessary because of all the modern controversies around the use of pharmacotherapy in the treatment of psychological disorders. The proponents of pharmacotherapy point to the "miraculous" development in the 1950s of the psychotropic medications, including chlorpromazine, lithium, and imipramine, and argue for their role in the reduced use of other treatments such as ECT and psychosurgery (see the next section), and the closure of the mental hospitals and the developments of community care. The opponents point to the medicalization of normal human misery by a pharmaceutical industry driven by an ever-increasing greed for profit, the less than impressive and often manipulated data on effectiveness, and the disabling side effects from the long-term use of psychotropic medication. The line that will be taken in this book is that perhaps there is a middle ground between these two extremes. In periods of high distress, many of us naturally turn to the short-term use of pharmaceuticals to help us get through, just as we might take a pain-killer for a bad headache or toothache, or vitamin D to get through the Scottish winter. Unfortunately, pharmacotherapy is heavily misused in psychiatry, with unnecessary long-term use and polypharmacy from cocktails of drugs because of non-response. A balanced approach to psychiatry has to offer social care, psychological support, and sometimes the possibility of short-term medication to help manage acute periods of distress. Members of all human societies have used naturally occurring psychotropic agents to alter how they feel, but our own predilection for such drugs has to be carefully managed in order to avoid irreversible longer-term damage from their use. This issue will be returned to in most of the chapters throughout this book, but next we will consider the development of psychosurgery as a form of psychiatric treatment.

Psychosurgery

Earlier we noted the archeological evidence that showed the use of trepanning, in which a hole is drilled into the skull in order to relieve "pressure" in the brain and to release demons from the skull. Removing the stone of folly, as it came to be known in the Middle Ages, consisted of trepanning carried out by peripatetic barber-surgeons, who at the same time could give you a nice haircut to match the hole in your head. The ancient procedure of trepanation seems only to have removed part of the skull, and it was not until the twentieth century that psychosurgery was added to the list of neuropsychiatric techniques. Of course, there had been famous cases such as that of Phineas Gage, the railroad worker who due to a blasting accident in 1848 had a large metal bar remove most of his frontal lobes, but the developers of psychosurgery should have noted that although Gage's basic cognitive functions were largely intact his personality changed for the worse and his socio-emotional skills deteriorated considerably (see, for example, the account in *Descartes' Error* by Antonio Damasio, 2005).

The first attempts at lobotomy, the cutting and separation of the frontal lobes from the rest of the brain, were carried out by the Swiss psychiatrist Gottlieb Burckhardt in 1888. Based on the simple theory that the brain consisted of sensory, motor, and "association" areas, Burckhardt reasoned that deletion of the association areas might lead to changes in functioning. He therefore operated on six patients suffering from chronic psychiatric illness; one of these died within a few days, two got worse, two remained the same, and one showed improvement. When he presented his results to his colleagues he met with considerable hostility and never repeated the procedure (Berrios, 1997). A variant of lobotomy, called leucotomy by its inventors, was developed by Anonio Egas Moniz and Pedro Lima in Lisbon in 1935. In leucotomy, rather than the whole lobe being separated from the rest of the brain a small loop of wire is rotated several times in each of the frontal lobes thereby disconnecting a series of small portions of the lobes. Over subsequent years different versions of leucotomy were developed, including electrocoagulation, in which a small electric current oblates the area of the brain between two electrodes, and yttrium-90 implants, in which radiation from the ^{90}Y isotope oblates the surrounding area. An estimated 40 000 lobotomies/leucotomies were carried out in the USA; one being on John F. Kennedy's sister Rose Kennedy, and 17 000 were carried out in the UK. In 1949, Moniz was controversially awarded Portugal's first Nobel Prize for the development of a procedure that deservedly fell into disrepute and has been banned in many countries. This was definitely one of the low points in the history of psychiatry, and was depicted as such in novels such as Ken Kesey's *One Flew Over the Cuckoo's Nest* (Kesey, 1962). This was made into a cult film in 1975 and includes a powerful performance by Jack Nicholson as the lead character who is lobotomized at the end of the film.

Hypnosis and Psychoanalysis

Franz Anton Mesmer (1734–1815) was so impressed by Isaac Newton's work on gravitational theory that he developed his own theory of "animal magnetism," which he believed to be a special force that acted between humans and other animals in the way that Newton's gravity acted between inanimate objects. Mesmer believed that animal magnetism was something that could aid in healing physical and mental disorders and he subsequently developed a large following in Parisian circles. Mesmer also believed that he possessed this animal magnetism in abundance, but his notoriety in Paris led to the French setting up a special Royal Commission in 1784 to investigate his claims (see Ellenberger, 1970). The commission included such notables as Benjamin Franklin (who was the American ambassador in Paris at the time), Antoine Lavoisier (a well-known chemist), and a certain Dr. Guillotin (who later became famous for an invention that was in frequent use during the French Revolution). Following their investigations the commission concluded that Mesmer's claims about animal magnetism were not true, but that nevertheless some of the people who attended Mesmer's individual or group sessions were helped through the "power of the imagination." Mesmer subsequently left Paris, and although the animal magnetism theory had been discredited a number Mesmer's followers continued to practice Mesmerism in Europe.

James Braid (1795–1860) was a Scottish physician who trained in Edinburgh but who practiced for most of his life in Manchester. Braid was influenced by the work of the Mesmerists but objected to what he saw as their exotic occult explanations for a phenomenon that could be understood in physiological and psychological terms. He therefore named the effect "hypnotism," the name by which the effect continues to be known. Braid's influence seems to have been greater in France than in Scotland or England, perhaps because the French had already proven more suggestible to Mesmerism. Subsequently, the most famous "hypnotist" of the nineteenth century was the French neurologist Jean-Martin Charcot (1825–93) who was professor at the Salpêtrière in Paris for 33 years. Charcot is seen by many as the founder of modern neurology, but he was also famous for his studies of hysteria and hypnosis that often included dramatic case presentations presented to packed audiences. Probably the most famous person to have attended Charcot's lectures was Sigmund Freud (1856–1939), who was present in Paris in October 1885. Freud was so inspired by Charcot's lectures that he returned to Vienna and abandoned his work in neurology in order to set up in private practice in 1886. He initially used hypnosis with his patients and worked in collaboration with his mentor Josef Breuer. However, one of his patients, Elizabeth von R, is reported to have been irritated by Freud's habit of interrupting her in order to hypnotize her every time she started talking about something interesting (see Gay, 1988). Freud stopped using hypnosis and switched to the method of free association, which he reported in his book written with Josef Breuer, *Studies on Hysteria*, first published in 1895.

An exploration of the background to and various developments of psychoanalysis is beyond the scope of the current book, though we will consider the impact of psychoanalysis on the development of psychotherapy and clinical psychology in the next section ("Clinical Psychology and Psychotherapy"). There have of course been many detractors from psychoanalysis and famous attacks on its proposals. However, many of these attacks, such as those of the philosopher Karl Popper (1963) who claimed that psychoanalysis is not falsifiable and is therefore not scientific, were based on ignorance or prejudice and have not been supported by later philosophical analyses (e.g., Grunbaum, 1984). The psychologist Hans Eysenck also claimed that psychoanalysis and psychodynamic therapies were not effective as treatments, a claim that we will consider in more detail next. As a tail note, however, we might add that the work of the psychoanalyst John Bowlby on attachment theory, which he developed in the 1950s, is having an increased impact on a range of areas such as child development, psychology, and psychotherapy.

Clinical Psychology and Psychotherapy

Although this chapter has focused primarily on psychiatry, the developments in clinical psychology and psychotherapy over the last 100 years have provided an important counterbalance to what many would see as an excessively medicalized approach to human suffering. Perhaps one of the least known "founding fathers/mothers" of any discipline has to be Lightner Witmer (1867–1956), who even most clinical psychologists have never heard of, never mind anyone from another discipline. Witmer was a doctoral student of Wilhelm Wundt, the founding father of experimental psychology, at his laboratory in Leipzig. Witmer then moved to the USA, where in 1896 at the University of Pennsylvania he opened a psychological clinic for children and coined the term "clinical psychology." The clinic offered a mix of research, training, evaluation, and child education.

Perhaps helped by Freud's visit to the USA in September 1909, psychoanalysis was very influential in the development of training courses in clinical psychology throughout that country, with many courses taking a strongly psychoanalytic approach, although contrary to Freud's wishes membership of the American Psychoanalytic Association was restricted to medical practitioners. In 1985 four psychologists filed a lawsuit against the association and its medical monopoly, which was settled in favor of the psychologists in 1988. We might note of course that some of the greatest contributions to psychoanalysis have come from its non-medical practitioners, including Anna Freud and Erik Erikson—another example of how medicine occasionally shoots itself in the foot, though at least it has now developed the techniques to save the foot even if it shot it in the first place!

By 1950 there were 149 graduate departments in the USA offering training in clinical psychology, including some that were teaching the new "Boulder scientist-practitioner" model developed by a group of clinical psychologists at a meeting in Boulder, Colorado in 1949. The scientist-practitioner model, with its scientific emphasis, tended to reflect the more behavioral approaches to psychology at that time, although subsequently it has become much broader as other approaches including the cognitive and the psychodynamic have been incorporated into the general scheme.

In contrast to the healthy position of clinical psychology in the USA, by 1950 clinical psychology in the UK consisted of a few psychometricians primarily carrying out assessments of IQ and personality but with no formal training in clinical psychology or in psychotherapy. Following his infamous attack on psychoanalysis in 1952, Hans Eysenck started the first UK training course at the Institute of Psychiatry in 1952, the famous 13-month Diploma in Abnormal Psychology that was headed by Monte Shapiro. Graduates from the course have contributed much over the years to the development of the psychotherapies, first to behavioral therapy but more recently to the cognitive-behavioral therapies.

It would be possible as we draw to the close of this race through a history of madness to be both prejudiced and simplistic and present psychiatrists as the bad guys in the treatment of madness with the new kids on the block, the clinical psychologists, as the good guys who have finally arrived to save the day. Just in case any medical readers are ready to point their fingers and say "What do you expect from a psychologist, anyway?!" I will mention some unacceptable and damaging procedures that have been used in the past in clinical psychology even given its brief history. When I started work at the Maudsley Hospital, London in the early 1980s, there was a group of mostly ex-patients who hung around Camberwell Green, to whom mention of the term "clinical psychology" was like a warning siren before an electrocution—literally. These unfortunate people had been under the "care" of clinical psychologists who tried to treat the "disorder" of homosexuality with aversion therapy, for example through the pairing of pictures of handsome men with electric shocks administered to the subject's genitals. We will return to the issue of the diagnosis of "disorders" such as homosexuality in Chapter 2, when we will examine it as an example of how the general approach to classification and diagnosis is fundamentally wrong. However, the point being made here is that it is not just medicine and psychiatry that have at times failed to preserve respect for and the dignity of those who have been labeled "mad"; even clinical psychology has fallen into the trap of developing "treatments" that have verged on the inhumane and are now illegal in many countries. Those that are the most vulnerable in society are also the most vulnerable to maltreatment and abuse by society itself, be they children, the elderly, or those labeled mad. Our treatments for madness must aim to alleviate suffering, not increase it.

2

DIAGNOSIS AND CLASSIFICATION

I can calculate the motion of heavenly bodies, but not the madness of people

Isaac Newton

Introduction

In this chapter we will examine some of the various and different approaches that have been used to classify and diagnose madness. Some of the historical background that has fed into the current classification systems will be briefly reviewed, but the current dominant systems, the American Psychiatric Association's Diagnostic and Statistical Manual (DSM) and the World Health Organization's International Classification of Diseases (ICD), will be looked at in most detail. There are of course a range of criticisms of these approaches to classification, and of the whole idea of classification itself—we will also consider the "case formulation" approach that has been promoted in clinical psychology and has been used as an alternative. In order to set classification in its true context, we will begin with a consideration of its uses within science, for example in chemistry.

Classification in Science

In Chapter 1 we considered some of the very early attempts at classification, such as the Greek concepts of the four elements and four humors and the Chinese system of five basic elements. These systems were ultimately shown to be flawed, or to be replaceable by more useful systems, but they are cited here as evidence that as humans we have a proclivity toward classifying that which we see around us, and of attempting to produce order out of chaos.

In chemistry, once it became clear that the ancient Greeks' "basic elements" of earth, air, fire, and water were divisible into a range of true elements, one of the challenges became the identification of exactly what those elements might be. For example, the English chemist Sir Humphry Davy, inventor of the miner's safety lamp, identified elements such as potassium, calcium, and magnesium; Antoine Lavoisier, the French chemist whom we met in Chapter 1 as a member of the Royal Commission that investigated Anton Mesmer, discovered that substances such as sulfur and chlorine were elements rather than compounds.

Such was the progress in chemistry that by the time that the great Russian chemist Dmitri Mendeleev, along with others, began to struggle with the possible classification of the chemical elements in the 1860s chemists already knew of 56 different chemical elements. Since then these numbers have more than doubled, to 118 at the last count (see Figure 2.1); however, it is worth making a short digression to recount the development of Mendeleev's periodic table, for within it there is a moral tale that has a bearing on psychiatry.

Mendeleev noticed that there were regular repeating patterns and similarities between different elements when they were ordered in terms of their atomic weights. Atomic weight was originally calculated from the average mass of one mole of the element relative to hydrogen, which was given a value of one (though the modern comparison is with carbon-12 rather than hydrogen). However, even Mendeleev was aware that classification based on atomic weight was flawed; for example, the elements tellurium and iodine occurred in the wrong order on the basis of their atomic weight, with iodine having a lower atomic weight but rightly having the properties of the halogen group (chlorine, fluorine, etc.) which tellurium does not. Mendeleev therefore decided to reverse the periodic sequence in their case. It was only in the twentieth century, when the structure of the atom based on protons and neutrons was identified, that the use of *atomic number* rather than *atomic weight* provided the ideal

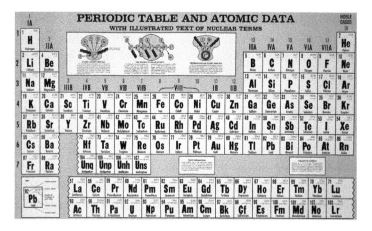

Fig. 2.1. Periodic table of the elements. © WidStock.

basis for the periodic table classification system. The atomic number of an element refers to its number of protons, which are the positively charged particles that are present in the atomic nucleus. However, the atomic nucleus also contains differing numbers of neutrons, neutral particles, within its structure. Because the chemical properties of an element are determined by the number of negatively charged electrons, which in the non-ionized form of the element matches the number of protons, there are many elements that have a number of *isotopes*, that is, have different numbers of neutrons, affecting the atomic weight but not the atomic number. Hence, Mendeleev's tellurium and iodine anomaly turned out to be because the tellurium he had sourced contained a preponderance of a heavier tellurium isotope giving it a greater atomic weight (based on the number of neutrons plus protons) than iodine, even though iodine has a higher atomic number (based on just protons alone).

Despite Mendeleev's initial system being flawed, and with the correct theoretical basis of the periodic table not being identified for another 50 years, Mendeleev was able to predict correctly a number of elements that had yet to be identified but which were expected to exist if the repeating periodic structure of the table was correct. These elements included gallium and germanium, whose properties Mendeleev had been able to outline because of their membership of the groups of poor metals that included known elements such as aluminum and silicon, respectively (hence Mendeleev's original names of "eka-aluminium" for gallium and "eka-silicon" for germanium). One of the great strengths of a theoretically based classification system, therefore, is that it can predict the existence of yet-to-be identified members of the system or can lead to a reclassification of members that have been misclassified under previous systems. The implications for psychiatric classification systems seem clear.

Griesinger, Kraepelin, Bleuler, and German Psychiatry

The real push toward classification in psychiatry came from German and to some extent French psychiatrists in the nineteenth century, with sporadic attempts in other countries such as Britain. Andrew Scull (e.g., Scull, 2011) has argued that whereas in the French- and English-speaking worlds psychiatry primarily had an administrative function within the nineteenth-century asylums, German psychiatry, in contrast, was integrated within the universities and research institutes. German psychiatrists therefore had far greater interest in understanding the possible etiology and taxonomy of the range of mental and physical conditions that affected mental functioning. The nineteenth century also witnessed considerable developments and advances in medicine more generally: these developments included the development of germ theory by scientists such as Louis Pasteur that replaced the earlier miasma or "bad air" theory of infectious disease; the cell theory developed by Theodor Schwann; and the application of cell theory to the neuron doctrine developed by Ramon y Cajal and Heinrich Waldeyer. These general medical developments had a strong influence on German psychiatry because psychiatry was incorporated into the research institutes and universities.

Wilhelm Griesinger (1817–68), who was originally a professor of medicine and infectious diseases in Tübingen then professor of pathology in Kiel, eventually moved to found the Burghölzli mental hospital in Zurich in 1860. There he established the German psychiatric tradition of the link between the clinic, the university, and the need for research rather than just management of the insane. He finally moved to Berlin where he was professor of psychiatry and head of the polyclinic. Griesinger's view was that mental illness was due to disease of the brain (e.g., Scull, 2011) and thereby set in motion the German tradition of careful examination of brain pathology and its links with mental illness. This movement of course had some notable successes; for example in 1906 Alois Alzheimer (1864–1915) identified plaques and tangles in the brain of a patient, Auguste Deter, whom he had first examined 5 years previously, thereby demonstrating the pathology and symptoms of presenile dementia. Although some of this information in relation to older adults and senile dementia had been known before Alzheimer's work (e.g., Berrios, 1995), Alzheimer's contribution was to show that such diseases can also occur in younger adults. Of course, this type of both presenile and senile dementia is now known as Alzheimer's disease, following the use of this label by Alzheimer's colleague Emil Kraepelin in the eighth edition of his *Handbook of Psychiatry* in 1910.

Kraepelin (1856–1926) was born in the same year as Sigmund Freud, which marks 1856 out as a remarkable year for the birth of those who were to become the fathers of modern psychiatry and psychoanalysis. He studied medicine in Leipzig and then moved to Würzburg, where he came under the influence of the founder of modern experimental psychology, Wilhelm Wundt (1832–1920), whose methods strongly influenced Kraepelin's approach to psychiatric research. Although now best remembered for his distinction between "dementia praecox" and "manic-depression," Kraepelin's work on classification is in fact far more sophisticated and has been a very strong influence on subsequent generations of psychiatric classifiers ever since. Kraepelin introduced the distinction between the endogenous psychoses of dementia praecox and manic-depression in the sixth edition of his textbook in 1899, in which dementia praecox was considered to be a progressive disease with a poor prognosis whereas manic-depression had a better prognosis. In 1899 he further distinguished three main types of dementia praecox as hebephrenic, catatonic, and paranoid forms, which was further expanded to 10 types in later editions, in addition to a broad range of disorders of personality. In 1911, the Swiss psychiatrist Eugen Bleuler (1857–1939), yet another great psychiatrist born just a year after Freud and Kraepelin, proposed that the term "dementia praecox" be replaced by the term "schizophrenia"; this reflected Bleuler's view that the disorder did not necessarily lead to a progressive deterioration and that it is better considered as a splitting between the emotional and intellectual functions. This was somewhat influenced by Freud's ideas on the unconscious, leading to more optimistic views on the possible outcome for schizophrenia. However, the notion of "splitting" has fed into a popular Hollywood-type view that mistakenly equates schizophrenia with a Jekyll and Hyde-type split personality that was never intended by Bleuler's use of the term (e.g., Turner, 1995), which refers to a splitting of the mind rather than of the personality.

One of the important criticisms of Kraepelin and his view of dementia praecox is the possibility that his patients were not those who would nowadays receive a diagnosis of schizophrenia; this is likely to have contributed to his view of the progressive deterioration that Bleuler and others subsequently challenged. One condition that contributed considerably to the number of nineteenth-century asylum inmates was syphilis of the central nervous system. For example, the great French psychiatrist Jean-Etienne Dominique Esquirol (1772–1840) had proposed the term "monomania" in the early 1800s; this could have a favorable outcome, but in a proportion of cases had an unfavorable outcome accompanied by paralysis. However, in 1822 another French psychiatrist, Antoine Bayle, published a disagreement with Esquirol, arguing for an organically caused *chronic arachnoiditis* in such cases (Berrios, 1995), which developed as a series of successive clinical syndromes. Bayle's disease was subsequently included under the wider term "general paralysis of the insane" (GPI), which Fournier in 1875 eventually proposed might be linked to syphilis. In 1858 Guillaume Duchenne also identified that another GPI-related disorder, *tabes dorsalis*, subsequently named Duchenne's disease in honor of his discovery, was also a consequence of syphilis. Estimations of the percentage of asylum admissions that were related to tertiary syphilis in the nineteenth century range from 10 to 29% (e.g., Scull, 2011). However, it was not until 1913 that the Japanese bacteriologist Hideyo Noguchi (1876–1928) working at the Rockefeller Institute in New York first demonstrated the presence of the syphilis spirochete in the brain of a GPI patient. Therefore one of the criticisms of nineteenth-century accounts of madness is that the common occurrence of conditions such as general paralysis was due to later-to-be discovered infections.

In her book *Schizophrenia: A Scientific Delusion*, Mary Boyle (2002) further extends the GPI-type criticism of Kraepelin's description of dementia praecox. As a number of later twentieth-century studies of schizophrenia have suggested, the presentation and severity of "schizophrenia" seem to have declined since the time of Kraepelin and

Bleuler (e.g., Der et al., 1990). Boyle suggests that "schizophrenia" populations in the late nineteenth and early twentieth centuries also included large numbers of patients who were suffering from encephalitis lethargica, mentioned in Chapter 1 (also known as Von Economo's disease after the doctor who first described it in 1917), many of whom went on to develop Parkinsonian-type symptoms. The population of Europe had been devastated by waves of epidemics of this disease and related flu epidemics, the best-known being the pandemic of Spanish flu shortly after the First World War, in which it is estimated more people died than in the war itself.

In summary, therefore, it seems possible that the "dementia praecox" identified by Kraepelin as a disease with progressive deterioration could have mistakenly included a number of other disorders such as GPI and encephalitic lethargica, plus a number of patients with Parkinson's disease and Huntington's disease who can sometimes present with similar symptoms. Bleuler's term "schizophrenia" soon replaced Kraepelin's term, in part because it did not imply such a pessimistic view of the course and outcome of the disorder, though even today many clinical psychiatrists still think of schizophrenia in more negative terms than manic-depressive disorders, in line with Kraepelin's proposals. However, given the problematic origins and history of the concept of "schizophrenia," perhaps it is now time to drop this diagnostic label altogether, as many of its recent critics have argued. We will return to this issue later in this chapter and in subsequent chapters.

A Note on Depression

The discussion so far on classification in psychiatry has focused on the problem of schizophrenia, but before we turn to the modern classification systems themselves it is worth pausing for a brief consideration of the term "depression."

The word "depression" derives from the Latin "deprimere," meaning "to push down." The use of the term was rare before the eighteenth century, but then it started to appear in everyday contexts, in part following the writings of Samuel Johnson who seems to have suffered from depression himself (see Jackson, 1986). The medical use of the term depression was introduced into psychiatry by influential nineteenth-century German practitioners such as Griesinger and Kraepelin, and has been largely incorporated into the modern psychiatric classification systems such as the DSM (American Psychiatric Association, 2013) and the ICD (World Health Organization, 1992). It should be noted, however, that the more common term from the time of Hippocrates until the nineteenth century had been "melancholia," deriving from the Greek for "black bile," one of the four humors; this term is still in occasional use today. Influential works such as Robert Burton's *The Anatomy of Melancholy* (Burton,

1621) and even Freud's *Mourning and Melancholia* (Freud, 1917) continued this usage, but it is extremely rare nowadays to see any formal mention of "melancholia" rather than "depression."

One of the enduring distinctions that has been made when trying to bring order to the heterogeneity of depression is between "unipolar" and "bipolar" depression. Recognition of the signs and symptoms of what we would now consider bipolar disorder dates back to Hippocrates and his associates in the fifth and fourth centuries BCE, who distinguished between mania and melancholia. The first description of it is credited to Aretaeus of Cappadocia (e.g., Porter, 1995), who stated in his books *The Treatment of Chronic Diseases* and *Symptomatology of Chronic Diseases* that "The development of mania is really a worsening of the disease [melancholia], rather than a change into another disease . . . In most of them [melancholics], the sadness became better after various lengths of time and changed into happiness; the patients then develop a mania." It was not until the advent of the German school of psychiatry that the classification of bipolar disorder advanced significantly. Kahlbaum's proposal that classifications of psychosis should consist of nosological entities signified a clearer conceptualization of mental illness. He put forward the concept of a close correspondence between clinical symptoms, course and outcome, cerebral pathology, and etiology as the criteria for correlated clinical states constituting a "natural disease entity." In using the phrase "cyclical insanity" he is also credited as the first person to refer to cyclothymia (Jauhar and Cavanagh, 2013). Kraepelin built on these suggestions with his division of the psychoses into manic-depressive insanity and dementia praecox, as we noted earlier, in which he held a unitary concept of manic-depressive illness.

Kraepelin's concept of manic-depressive illness has been described in terms of excitement or inhibition (increase or decrease) of three basic areas: mood, thinking, and activity. All three can move in a coordinated direction, leading to episodes of mania, hypomania, or depression; or they can move in opposite directions, resulting in mixed states, defined as combinations of manic or hypomanic and depressive symptoms in the same episode. Crucially, mood did not have to be increased for a diagnosis of mania to be made (the other two symptoms of activity and thinking could be increased). An emphasis was placed on *recurrence*, family history, episodic course (episodes including mixed states, recurrent depression, hypomania, or mania), and young age of onset (Jauhar and Cavanagh, 2013).

Although better known for his contribution to the classification of schizophrenia, the Swiss psychiatrist Eugen Bleuler also played a part in the modern classification of bipolar disorder, broadening manic-depressive insanity into categories of affective illness (see Goodwin and Jamison, 2007). The psychiatrists Karl Leonhard and Carlo Perris then took this further, proposing the distinction between unipolar and bipolar depression, one that continues into the current DSM and ICD classification systems, as we will discuss subsequently. In 1980 the term bipolar disorder replaced that of manic-depressive disorder in DSM-III, reflecting the observation, contrary to the earlier German view, that not all of those with the disorder went on to develop psychosis, which further differentiated the disorder from schizophrenia.

The DSM and ICD Systems of Classification

The American Psychiatric Association (APA) enterprise to classify and diagnose mental disorders began systematically with the publication of the first DSM in 1952. The APA drew on the World Health Organization's (WHO) ICD system (or the International Classification of Diseases, Injuries and Causes of Death, as it was then called), which by 1952 was in its sixth edition, published in 1949 just after the founding of the WHO. The ICD included all known diseases along with a range of psychiatric disorders, and had originated in the work of Farr and D'Espine, who in 1853 had been asked by the International Statistical Congress to produce an agreed list of the causes of death, known as the International List of Causes of Death. The ICD was originally designed simply to facilitate the recording of data on causes of death, but after 1949 also on the prevalence of all known diseases, while the DSM had a somewhat different aim from its initiation. The ICD classification listed the names of diseases and their subtypes, but the DSM system attempted to provide "working definitions or thumbnail descriptions of the syndromes concerned" (Kendell, 1975, p. 92).

The first version of DSM, DSM-I, had a total of 128 pages and 106 diagnoses. By the time of the second revision, DSM-II, in 1968, there were 134 pages and 182 diagnoses. The third revision, DSM-III, in 1980 had 494 pages and 265 diagnoses; its revision DSM-III-R appeared in 1987 with 567 pages and 292 diagnoses. The fourth revision, DSM-IV, appeared in 1994 and contained 886 pages with 365 diagnoses (a different diagnosis for every day of the year), with a text revision DSM-IV-TR appearing in 2000 with 943 pages. We will save commentary on DSM-5, which was published in 2013, until the next section. This diagnostic inflation across the versions of the DSM has been heavily criticized, even by leading contributors to the DSM such as Allen Frances (2013).

The general methodology for the DSM revisions is worth spelling out, especially given the tendency to increase the number of diagnostic categories with each revision. In contrast to the theoretical scientifically based systems in chemistry mentioned earlier, the approach taken with DSM is atheoretical and relies instead on expert consensus. As Robert Spitzer (1991) stated about the DSM-III revision, for which he was the chair, the committee would have been unable to include over 200 of the diagnoses if scientific evidence had been required for their inclusion.

The DSM-IV Task Force was chaired by Allen Frances and consisted of 13 work groups, a committee on assessment, and the APA Board of Trustees who made the final decisions on the recommendations from the Task Force (Frances, 2013). Over 1000 individuals were involved in one way or another with the DSM-IV revision of 1994. Mindful of the adage "a camel is a horse designed by a committee," the first question that has to be asked is why 13 work groups? Whose lucky number does that reflect? Appendix J of DSM-IV (1994) details each of the work groups together with their membership. For example, the Anxiety Disorders Work Group consisted of six people chaired by Michael Liebowitz, but drew on advice from 108 additional named individuals. The Premenstrual Dysphoric Disorder Work Group consisted of six people chaired by Judith Gould, which drew on advice from 36 additional named individuals. Hang on, you mean there really was a whole group that considered a proposed single diagnostic category of premenstrual dysphoric disorder? The existence of such groups reflects little or nothing of science but simply the power of one or more individuals to influence the proceedings of a committee and get their name attached to a new "syndrome." In the end, premenstrual dysphoric disorder was not given full diagnostic status but was relegated to Appendix B in DSM-IV, which included a number of other "needs further study" diagnoses such as "mixed anxiety-depressive disorder," "factitious disorder by proxy" (sometimes known in Europe controversially as "Munchausen syndrome by proxy," named after the German Baron von Münchhausen [sic.] who was famous for his exaggerated tall stories), and "postconcussional disorder."

Let us examine the DSM-IV work group proposals and decisions about the anxiety disorders. The first point we need to make, and one that will be returned to in later chapters, is why does the basic emotion of anxiety have a whole chapter to itself with numerous disorders, yet the basic emotion of *anger* does not even appear in the index for DSM-IV let alone have any diagnostic categories? Surely in the history of *Homo sapiens* anger disorders have been far more dysfunctional and destructive than anxiety disorders? Somebody, presumably Allen Frances the Task Force chair and his more than 1000 advisers, forgot to create a work group to consider anger disorders. Had they done so, presumably we would by now have a whole bucket load of such disorders. This problem is just the first of many that occur when classification is done by committee consensus rather than by theoretical understanding.

The second problem that arises is a type of in-group/out-group phenomenon, well known in social psychology (e.g., Tajfel and Turner, 1979), in which the group presumes that because it has been handed phenomena like phobias, compulsions, and post-trauma reactions to classify they must therefore be *anxiety disorders*. Similarly, because it has not been handed phenomena like somatoform, dissociative, and adjustment disorders, because they all fell under the aegis of another work group to classify, they therefore must not be anxiety disorders. Take the example of post-traumatic stress disorder (PTSD; category 309.81), which is listed in DSM-IV as an anxiety disorder in which the experience of a severe trauma is accompanied by a number of re-experiencing (e.g., intrusive images, distressing dreams, and feelings of recurrence), avoidance, and hyper-arousal symptoms. However, we know from both theoretical and clinical analyses of PTSD (Dalgleish and Power, 2004) and studies of the prevalent emotions in PTSD (Power and Fyvie, 2013) that only in about 50% of cases that meet DSM-IV diagnostic criteria for PTSD is anxiety the most prevalent emotion; in the other 50% the emotions of anger, disgust, or sadness may be more predominant than anxiety. So why therefore is PTSD listed as an *anxiety disorder* when the predominant emotion need not be anxiety? In fact, similar problems arise with certain types of phobia and obsessive compulsive disorder (OCD) which are listed as anxiety disorders, some of which may be predominantly disgust-based reactions rather than anxiety-based reactions (Power and Dalgleish, 2008). We will return to this issue in the next section when we consider the revisions for the current DSM-5, which has taken on board many of these criticisms.

DSM-IV also continued an innovation that had started in DSM-III in the form of a *multi-axial assessment*, i.e., the idea that an individual could receive ratings on each of the following five dimensions:

Axis I: clinical disorders
Axis II: personality disorders; mental retardation (as it was called in the USA)
Axis III: general medical conditions
Axis IV: psychosocial and environmental problems
Axis V: global assessment of functioning.

The aim of the multi-axial system was to provide more of a bio-psychosocial context in which the clinical and personality disorders could be described. In practice, clinicians and researchers primarily used axes I and II, with rarer use of the other axes except for some typically separate use of the global assessment of functioning (GAF) 1–100 rating scale. The fact that the multi-axial system was nice in theory but little used in practice seems to have contributed to its demise, because it has been abandoned in DSM-5 (see the next section, "DSM-5").

Before we go on to consider the development of DSM-5, it is worth looking at DSM-III (American Psychiatric Association, 1980) in more detail because it is considered as the landmark development in the history of the DSMs. The chair of the Task Force was Robert Spitzer, Professor at the New York State Psychiatric Unit, Columbia University, who is now considered by many to be one of the most influential psychiatrists of the twentieth century. The previous versions of DSM had in part reflected the strong psychoanalytic influence on American psychiatry; however, the accompanying diagnostic categories were often complex and extremely unreliable in their use. The study of psychometrics tells us that if you do not have reliability in the measurement of a concept then you certainly cannot have validity (e.g., Cronbach, 1967). One of Spitzer's main aims therefore was to increase diagnostic reliability through the specification of diagnostic criteria; thus, previous editions of DSM and ICD assumed that clinicians and researchers simply knew from their experience what these criteria were. However, the famous WHO study, *The International Pilot Study of* Schizophrenia (World Health Organization 1973), had compared the incidence and diagnosis of schizophrenia in several different countries. It included and supported conclusions from an earlier US–UK diagnostic study (e.g., Cooper et al., 1972) that American psychiatrists were more likely than their British colleagues to diagnose schizophrenia as opposed to manic-depression in their patients. DSM-III therefore set out to establish reliable diagnostic criteria for each of its proposed diagnoses. In his account of the development of DSM-III in his book *What is Mental Illness?* Richard McNally recounts behind-the-scenes DSM stories such as the following:

> One iconic image depicts Robert Spitzer and his neo-Kraepelinian colleagues sitting around a table, formulating new diagnostic categories on the spot, while Spitzer taps out the defining criteria on his typewriter (McNally 2011, p. 33).

Of course, as we noted earlier, Spitzer himself stated that although his aim was to provide scientific support for the diagnostic categories through the specification of reliable diagnostic criteria, most diagnoses did not have such criteria available. Research psychiatry has subsequently set out to collect such reliable diagnostic criteria and we will attempt to come to a judgment on its success or otherwise when we review the latest offerings in DSM-5. Before we do so, however, we will provide a brief comment on what happens to the camel (a horse designed by a committee) with the example of the original inclusion and subsequent exclusion of "homosexuality" as a diagnostic category.

The problem for the earlier versions of the DSM was that Freud had viewed homosexuality as problematic, so that the strong influence of psychoanalysis on American psychiatry was reflected in the inclusion of homosexuality as a diagnostic category. In works such as *Three Essays on the Theory of Sexuality*, Freud (1905) viewed homosexuality as an inversion of normal sexual development. The first DSM in 1952 therefore considered sexual pathological behavior as a category that included "pathological behavior, such as homosexuality, transvestism, pedophilia, fetishism, and sexual sadism, including rape, sexual assault, mutilation." However, the 1960s and 1970s witnessed important social changes with movements toward societal acceptance of homosexuality rather than its pathologization. Here we meet Robert Spitzer again, chair of the Task Force for the DSM-III revision, who during one of the APA meetings was confronted by a gay rights demonstration. Spitzer then secretly attended a gay psychiatry meeting and was apparently surprised by how many intelligent healthy seeming psychiatrists were there! Under his stewardship, therefore, homosexuality was subsequently eliminated from DSM-III as a diagnostic category following a democratic vote of the members of the APA. As a tail note though, Spitzer was later to get into trouble with the gay community with a paper published in 2003 in the *Archives of Sexual Behavior* in which he suggested that many of them could benefit from "reparative therapy" that could switch them back to heterosexuality. Following an onslaught of criticism of both the proposal and the flawed research behind it, Spitzer has apparently tried to retract the paper from the journal, but the journal editor has refused to allow its retraction. The problem for sexual orientations and practices such as homosexuality is that they are often defined as "non-normative," but if any classification system includes some aspect of population norms in its definitions, then a whole range of sexual practices including the "paraphilias" (sexual arousal to non-normative objects) become defined as pathological. If, for example, a man finds it sexually arousing to wear a skirt or a dress, why should that reflect any form of pathology? In fact, I live in a country, Scotland, where men do exactly that as part of their national costume. The equivalent argument would be that because some heterosexuals are rapists, *heterosexuality* should therefore be made into a disorder. The problem lies with the clinical method and fallacious induction from individual cases—that because one homosexual has problems homosexuality is therefore a problem (one swan is white, therefore all swans are white).

DSM-5

The latest revision of the DSM, DSM-5, was published in May 2013 after 14 years in the making. The first trivial question to ask is why have the APA switched from Roman numerals (DSMs I–IV) to Arabic numerals (DSM-5)? The answer is not that the Task Force did not know what the Roman numeral for five was, but that apparently in the electronic age Roman numerals do not work as well as Arabic ones.

The chair of the DSM-5 Task Force, David Kupfer, again went for 13 work groups with 8 to 15 members per group, though the Premenstrual Dysphoric Disorder Work Group from DSM-IV clearly did not get the vote and so was not reconvened. Instead, the most obvious new work group that reflects pressure and "current fashion" in diagnosis has to be the ADHD [attention deficit hyperactivity disorder] and Disruptive Behavior Disorders Work Group chaired by David Shaffer. On the positive side, DSM-5 has broken the trend of past DSMs by not adding excessively to the number of diagnostic categories but instead has gone for revising and restructuring many of the existing categories. For example, we raised the issue above about the incorrect placement of PTSD within the anxiety disorders because in approximately 50% of cases an emotion other than anxiety such as anger, disgust, or sadness seems to be predominant in the reaction to trauma (Power and Fyvie, 2013). The revision in DSM-5 has been to place PTSD in its own stand-alone category (in a chapter named "Trauma- and stressor-related disorders"). A similar problem with OCD, i.e., that only some types of OCD seem to be anxiety based but others seem to be disgust based, has also led to OCD being removed from under the anxiety disorders umbrella and placed in its own category.

A behind-the-scenes look at the in-fighting in DSM-5 over personality disorders would have been well worth buying a ticket for. The personality disorders were given a separate axis within DSM-IV, in which they were placed on Axis II, but the multi-axial approach first introduced in DSM-III has been abandoned in DSM-5 with the justification that people could always receive multiple diagnoses anyway so there was no need for a separate axis for the personality disorders. More interestingly, we have recently published (Emmelkamp and Power, 2012) some articles from members of the DSM-5 Personality Disorders Work Group, two of whom (John Livesley and Roel Verhuel) stepped down in 2012 before the work group had completed its task because of irreconcilable disagreements within the group. Personality and personality disorders have always provided some of the most fraught issues for the DSM task forces to deal with, in part because of the extreme positions between those who propose dimensional approaches and those who prefer categorical approaches, and in part because the personality disorder categories have been very vulnerable to prevailing fashions. For example, there were 12 personality disorders in DSM-I (1952), that included inadequate and passive–aggressive personality disorders, DSM-II (1968) had 10 types including explosive and asthenic, DSM-III (1980) had 11 types that included histrionic and narcissistic, and DSM-IV (1994) had 10 types with the passive–aggressive, self-defeating, and sadistic types now being dropped (see Coolidge and Segal, 1998, for a summary). Up until DSM-IV, therefore, the work in personality psychology, which was primarily based on dimensions, had mostly been ignored. In contrast, however, the plan for DSM-5 was that finally the two major approaches, the categorical and the dimensional, would be combined by the Personality Disorders Work Group. The problem was that the work group failed to reach agreement on how the dimensions and categories could be brought together, which led to Livesley and Verhuel stepping down in disagreement with the committee. We were therefore forced to make the recommendation that the task force should abandon the attempt to combine the contrasting approaches because of the lack of agreement (Emmelkamp and Power, 2012), a recommendation that the DSM-5 group has subsequently accepted. However, the personality group for the revised ICD-11, likely to be published in 2016, has returned to the attempt and seems likely to approve a much-simplified dimensional approach.

The behind-the-scenes fall-outs on the DSM Personality Disorders Work Group are symptomatic of what happens when classification systems are based on so-called consensus agreements of hundreds of experts rather than on scientific theory. In consensus approaches it is typically the alpha male with the highest status who shouts the loudest who wins the classification battle. For example, it might seem like a victory for science that OCD and PTSD have been extracted from the anxiety disorders category on the basis of the empirical evidence that has accumulated to the contrary. However, these stand-alone categories now simply group together disorders that are based on different basic emotions (see Chapter 3), which might or might not be warranted. What if the disgust-based reactions, be they traumatic, compulsive, obsessional, or phobic, are more similar to each other than they are to anxiety-based or anger-based reactions that DSM-5 lumps together? These and other related issues will form the focus of subsequent chapters, but before we turn to these issues, in the remainder of this chapter we will consider some of the attempts that have been made to look at different possible theoretical underpinnings for the classification of disorders, and we will also examine some of the medico-legal issues that are raised by the concept of madness.

Other Approaches to Psychiatric Classification

The DSM claim that it is *atheoretical* (and proud of it!) is of course unlikely to be true, because theories have implicit effects on our reasoning and decision-making even if we disavow their existence (Kahneman, 2011). A careful review of the history and development of the DSMs reveals a series of theoretical influences that have waxed and waned over the years, including the psychoanalytic, the behavioral, the cognitive, and the neuroscientific. However, there have been some attempts to at least group together the psychiatric diagnoses according to meaningful systems, even if the theoretical and etiological bases of the nosologies have not been spelled out, or the systems are partial rather than complete accounts of possible psychiatric diagnostic categories. In this section, we will examine hierarchical approaches to classification, beginning with the model put forward by Graham Foulds and Alan Bedford (Foulds and Bedford, 1975; Foulds, 1976). We will then consider the dimensional approach to some of the emotional disorders that has been considered in the work of David Watson and Lee Anna Clark (e.g., Watson and Clark, 1992).

The Foulds and Bedford (1975) hierarchical model argued that the diagnostic systems typically fail to make statements about the relative ordering of diagnoses against each other, or only make such orders implicit when such hierarchical ordering should be explicit. They proposed the following four overarching categories:

1. Dysthymic states: changes in affect that are common to all psychiatric states.
2. Neurotic symptoms: examples include dissociation, fear, rumination, and compulsions that are experienced as alien to the normal self.
3. Integrated delusions: delusions of persecution, delusions of grandeur, etc.
4. Delusions of disintegration: for example paranoia where the sense of self has disintegrated.

These four classes form a hierarchical pyramid, with the rarest category (4) at the top, then category (3), then (2), with category (1), the dysthymic states, at the bottom. One of the consequences of a hierarchical ordering is that if the person has symptoms at a higher level of the hierarchy the presence of symptoms at all lower levels is implied; for example, if the person has a delusion of grandeur, this rarer symptom will be accompanied by lower-level symptoms such as fear and rumination at the neurotic symptom level and a range of changes in affect at the lowest dysthymic states level. Foulds and Bedford developed the Delusions–Symptoms–States Inventory (DSSI), which they used to test their hierarchical model. Their analysis of 480 patients from a range of English, Scottish, and Canadian hospitals showed that 93.3% of the cases conformed to their hierarchical model. Furthermore, when using the hierarchical model they found that 58% of the patients were assigned to a single syndrome within the model.

In a study that used the Present State Examination (PSE; Wing et al., 1974) rather than the DSSI, Elizabeth Sturt (1981) reported on the hierarchical organization within diagnoses in data collected from several samples of inpatients, outpatients, and community participants. Sturt reported partial support for the Foulds and Bedford model, but found that a variant of the hierarchy with schizophrenia at the top, then other psychotic, then specific neurotic, then non-specific neurotic fitted the data even better. Sturt's analyses showed that the rarer symptoms such as the psychotic ones were typically associated with more of the lower-level neurotic symptoms, but the hierarchical model did not have to be the specific one detailed by Foulds and Bedford. Further studies showed that patients with more long-standing problems did not fit the Foulds and Bedford hierarchy as well as newer patients did (McGorry, 1994). Bagshaw and McPherson (1978) also found that a group of manic and hypomanic patients did not fit the model well.

Dimensional Approaches

As noted earlier, there are dimensional as well as categorical approaches to areas such as emotion and personality. Although the dimensional approaches are very influential in the area of normal psychology, attempts to incorporate them into the DSM classification system for personality disorders have so far been fraught with difficulty and seem to have been postponed until at least DSM-6, ICD-11, and beyond (Emmelkamp and Power, 2012). In this subsection, therefore, we will focus on dimensional approaches to the emotions and how these have been used to provide a partial classification system for at least some of the emotional disorders, even though they have not been applied to all psychological disorders.

There have been long-standing proposals about whether or not emotions are best characterized by specific dimensions or by discrete emotional categories. Dimensions such as that of the importance of pleasure versus pain can be traced back to Plato, to Spinoza, to Wundt, and to Freud, whereas proposals for discrete emotional categories are most clearly presented in the work of Descartes and Darwin. There have been several related proposals since the 1950s that have focused on dimensions such as valence and arousal. Osgood's work on the "semantic differential" identified dimensions related to arousal and valence in factors that consistently emerged from ratings of verbal and pictorial mood- and emotion-related stimuli (e.g., Osgood et al., 1957). The importance of the arousal component was later highlighted in one of the key early psychological theories of emotion, that of Schachter and Singer (1962). Later theories have divided up the dimensions of valence and arousal somewhat differently. Gray (e.g., Gray 1982) argued that the arousal system is in fact two separate systems that he labeled the behavioral activation system and the behavioral inhibition system, with overactivity and/or underactivity in either leading to different emotional consequences (see Power, 2005, for a critique). In contrast, Watson et al. (1988) have argued that the valence dimension, which is normally labeled with positive and negative as bipolar opposites, should be divided into two separate orthogonal dimensions one of which is positive and the other of which is negative. This proposal has attracted strong criticism from Russell and Carroll (1999), to the degree that the original authors are at least wavering in their views (Watson and Tellegen, 1999).

An emotion that is frequently observed along with depression is that of anxiety; thus, self-report measures of depression and anxiety typically correlate at about 0.7 across a range of populations (Clark and Watson, 1991; Goldberg and Goodyer, 2005). Indeed, the so-called tripartite model proposed by Clark and Watson (1991) and Clark (2000) argues that there is a common core of "negative affect" that forms the major component of a range of emotions including depression and anxiety. While there is much to be commended in such analyses, we take issue with the basic underlying model: first, because so-called negative affects are not necessarily experienced as negative, as we have argued elsewhere (Power and Dalgleish, 2008); second, because most of the results are based on student populations or, even in their tests of the model, patient groups such as those with drug problems that do not directly test the model (Watson et al., 1995a,b); and, third, because individuals may show less anxiety rather than more as they become increasingly depressed (Peterson et al., 1993). We would therefore concur for once with the decision of DSM-IV (American Psychiatric Association, 1994) that more evidence is necessary before the putative category of mixed anxiety–depression can be introduced. These points do not in any way deny the high comorbidity of depression and anxiety, particularly for less severe depression, and, indeed, there is every likelihood that the coupling together of the basic emotions involved in depression together with anxiety will undoubtedly lead to a prolongation of this distressing state. However, the proposal is that anxiety is not a defining feature of depression, nor depression of anxiety. What we do wish to emphasize is that severe life events often unfold over time rather than occur suddenly and out of the blue, they often occur in the context of related long-term difficulties (e.g., Brown et al., 1995), and in depression-prone individuals they can occur in an over-invested domain about which there is already considerable worry (Champion and Power, 1995). In addition, the threat of loss may subsequently turn into an actual loss, and so a state of anxiety in which the individual remains hopeful may turn into a state of depression in which the individual feels hopeless (Alloy et al., 2006).

In summary, in areas such as the emotions and personality dimensional approaches have been applied with some success to normal emotion and normal personality, but their application to the diagnostic and classification systems, while strongly supported by many, has yet to be satisfactorily accomplished. Our argument, however, is that such an endeavor cannot be successful while the dimensional approaches are based on psychological theories but the classification systems remain atheoretical. Mixing chalk and cheese will not work; thus, the answer has to lie with a common theoretical basis for both the dimensions and the categories before the two approaches can be successfully combined in the way that they have been in theoretical physics in the form of waves and particles.

Legal Approaches to Madness

Daniel M'Naghten (1813–65; properly "McNaughtan" but misspelled at the time of his trial) was a Scottish woodworker, sometime actor, and political activist who on the afternoon of January 20, 1843 walked up behind Edward Drummond, the then prime minister's secretary, as he was walking in London along Whitehall toward Downing Street, and shot him in the back at point blank range. Drummond died 5 days later, though perhaps as much from his treatment, which included bloodletting and leeches, as from the gunshot wound. It is thought that M'Naghten believed that he had actually shot the British prime minister, Robert Peel, himself rather than his secretary. M'Naghten was suffering from paranoid delusions that the Tories were persecuting him and pursuing him with their spies, and his defense team argued that he was "not guilty by reason of insanity." The case was used therefore by the House of Lords to spell out the legal insanity rules, with a special panel set up at the Old Bailey and chaired by Chief Justice Sir Nicholas Tindal. These rules are still in use today, albeit in adapted form, in many jurisdictions throughout the world and they became known as the "M'Naghten rules." M'Naghten himself spent the next 21 years of his life in the Bethlem Hospital before being moved to the newly opened Broadmoor Asylum in 1864, where he died the following year.

John Hinckley Junior was born in Oklahoma in 1955. He became obsessed with the film *Taxi Driver*, in which Robert de Niro plays Travis Bickle, a Vietnam veteran who attempts to shoot a US senator but who inadvertently becomes a hero because of his attempts to save Iris, a 12-year-old street prostitute played by Jodie Foster. After seeing the film, Hinckley became obsessed with Jodie Foster and eventually even took a writing course at Yale University where she was a student at the time. However, Foster rejected Hinckley's letters, phone calls, and poems, so, and inspired by the plot of *Taxi Driver*, he devised a plan for the "greatest love offering in the history of the world" by attempting on Monday March 30, 1981 to assassinate the newly elected president, Ronald Reagan. At his trial, Hinckley was found not guilty by reason of insanity and was given a diagnosis of schizophrenia and committed to St. Elizabeth's Hospital in Washington. There would also seem to be the issue of de Clerambault's syndrome (erotomania) in the nature of his obsession with Jodie Foster.

The two well-known cases of M'Naghten and Hinckley highlight a legal aspect of classification and diagnosis through the question of under what conditions or circumstances the "not guilty by reason of insanity" defense might be applied. Of course, different jurisdictions have developed different precedents on this question. For example, some jurisdictions include a type of "temporary insanity," or in France the *crime passionnel*, defense. In such states, the person becomes so overwhelmed by powerful emotions such as rage or jealousy that they are deemed no longer responsible for their actions, in which they may murder someone but without any prior premeditation. The crime of passion defense of temporary insanity was first used in the USA by Congressman Daniel Sickles of New York in 1859. Sickles claimed that he was driven out of his mind when he discovered that his young wife was having an affair with Philip Barton Key, whom he subsequently shot and killed.

The insanity defense requires both actus reus (that the defendant committed the unlawful act) and also mens rea, a Latin phrase that translates as "guilty mind," but given the possible absence of feelings of guilt, in modern law refers to "malice aforethought," that the defendant acted with knowledge and intention of the possible consequences of the act. The capacity of mens rea may be compromised by four factors that can be taken into account:

1. Age: for example, under the age of 10 in England and under age of 12 (previously age 8) in Scotland children are not considered criminally responsible for their acts.

2. Mental disorder: not only that the defendant would have received a diagnosis such as of schizophrenia or depression at the time of the act, but that the condition caused a defect of reason, and therefore the capacity to know that the act was wrong was absent at the time the act was committed.

3. The effects of drugs or alcohol: usually only usable if there are "disease of the mind"-type complications from the use of alcohol or drugs, rather than mere intoxication itself.

4. Automatism: an *insane automatism* is when an act is a consequence of a disease of the mind, but a *non-insane automatism* does not involve a disease of the mind and has even included proof of absent-mindedness leading to acquittal from a shoplifting offence.

A further Scottish innovation from 1867 is the concept of *diminished responsibility*, subsequently introduced into other jurisdictions, which permits some of the uncertainty about clear-cut judgments of an absence of mens rea at the time of an act to be taken into consideration, such that diminished responsibility is now applied in almost all convictions for murder where the insanity defense is accepted (e.g., Chiswick, 1998).

In summary, the legal requirements for the insanity defense require an interesting mix of retrospective diagnosis (i.e., the likely diagnosis at the time of the actus reus) and the current diagnosis (which may impact on fitness-to-plead judgments) with the additional requirements for mens rea that are only clear-cut in the case of age of the defendant (though this age varies across jurisdictions; for example, in different US states it ranges from 6 to 12 years; in Iran it is 9 for girls and 15 for boys; in Peru it is 18). Given how difficult it often is for clinicians to reach consensus on a *current* diagnosis, the need for a retrospective diagnosis plus judgment of mens rea can be fraught with difficulty. As an example of how difficult these decisions are in practice, we will consider the recent case in Norway of Anders Breivik, and the contradictory steps that the medico-legal process went through in an attempt to reach a verdict.

Anders Breivik

Anders Breivik was born on February 13, 1979 in Oslo. His mother, Wenche, worked as a nurse, and his father Jens was an economist and diplomat. His parents divorced when he was 18 months old, and although his father fought for custody, Anders lived with his mother. By the age of 4 there were already concerns about the young Breivik, with a psychiatric report expressing concern about the mother–son relationship, which was described as sexualized and overly aggressive (see Orange, 2012, *The Mind of a Madman: Norway's Struggle to Understand Anders Breivik*). At the time, his mother was described as depressed and personality disordered. She subsequently remarried an army officer, but Breivik seems to have had mixed views about his new stepfather, veering from describing him as a nice guy to, more memorably, referring to him as "a very primitive sexual beast." Breivik was confirmed as a Lutheran aged 15 and later joined the St. Olaf's Masonic Lodge in Oslo, which seems to have encouraged an interest in the Knights Templar and the supposed links between them and the Freemasons. He attended school in Oslo including the Ris Junior High School, and then studied at the Oslo School of Commerce. Friends from that time described him as intelligent and physically stronger than his classmates because of his regular weight training and his use of anabolic steroids, and they said that he had helped classmates who were bullied. Nevertheless, he was deemed unfit for military service and so was exempt from conscription to the Norwegian army. As a young adult Breivik worked in customer relations in a firm in Oslo, but then set up a number of his own companies including a computer programming company. Sometime in the spring of 2011 he moved to a farm in Hedmark to the northeast of Oslo. His supposed interest in farming seems to have been a cover that allowed him to buy fertilizer and experiment with explosives.

On Friday July 22, 2011 Breivik parked a car containing approximately 950 kg of a fertilizer-based explosive in front of Norwegian government buildings in Oslo, and detonated the explosive at 15.25. The explosion killed 8 people and injured a further 209. Next, he drove to the small island of Utoya, 25 miles from Oslo, where less than 2 hours later he landed from the small ferry boat that went to the island. The island that day, and for several days that week, was playing host to the Norwegian Labour Party's summer youth camp. Breivik was dressed in police uniform when he landed. He first killed the camp leader and the security officer who came to see him when he got off the ferry, having told them that he had been sent to increase security on the island following the attack in Oslo. Over the next one-and-a-half hours he hunted down and killed a total of 69 people, mostly teenagers, and injured another 110 people on the island. Eventually a police SWAT team arrived and he surrendered without further violence or attempts to resist arrest at 18.35.

Breivik was subsequently taken to Norway's Ila Prison, where he has been detained for most of the time since his arrest. Two forensic psychiatrists, Torgeir Husby and Synne Sorheim, were given the task of producing a psychiatric report on Breivik. Over the following weeks, they interviewed him 13 times and concluded that he suffered from the ICD-10 diagnosis of paranoid schizophrenia, F20.0. The main reasons they gave in support of their diagnosis were his blunted affect, the use of neologisms (new words or phrases of his own invention such as "cultural Marxists" and "national Darwinists"), and the presence of a delusional system that included the fictitious Knights Templar organization of the "Justiciar Knights," of which he was the Grand Master. Breivik's stated aim was to clear Europe of the "Eurabia conspiracy" (a conspiratorial belief among some extreme right-wing activists that there is a Muslim plan to take over Europe), through the elimination of the left-wing Marxists who were part of the conspiracy. These beliefs were spelled out in a 1518-page manifesto "2083: A European Declaration of Independence," which he had circulated on the internet shortly before the attacks. When asked why he had chosen Friday July 22 to go to Utoya, he stated that he thought that the former Norwegian prime minister and ex-head of the WHO, Gro Harlem Brundtland, would be visiting the island that day. Although Gro Harlem Brundtland was often referred to in Norwegian as the "Landsmoderen" (mother of the nation), Breivik referred to her as the "Landsmorderen" (murderer of the nation) instead (Orange, 2012). His plan was to capture Brundtland and then film a ritual beheading of her, Al-Qaeda style, but she had already left the island shortly before Breivik arrived.

The first psychiatric report from Husby and Sorheim was leaked to the press almost immediately on its completion on November 29, 2011 (it is available online at <https://sites.google.com/site/breivikreport/>, accessed May 20, 2013). Two experts, Svenn Torgersen, a professor of clinical psychology in Oslo, and Randi Rosenqvist, a leading Norwegian forensic psychiatrist, criticized the report immediately on its release in the media, stating that Breivik's actions had been too well planned and too well coordinated over a long period of time for him to be given a diagnosis of schizophrenia. There followed a national outcry against the psychiatric diagnosis, because in Norwegian law such a diagnosis would mean that Breivik was not criminally responsible whether or not there was mens rea at the time of the criminal action, and there is always the perception that the "criminally insane" verdict somehow lets criminals off their crimes, even though they can be detained in a psychiatric facility in perpetuity. However, Breivik himself seems to have been appalled that he might be declared criminally insane, and he rejected the first psychiatric report as "the ultimate humiliation." He wanted to be declared sane and have his acts seen as those of a revolutionary leader, but he realized that his manifesto and actions might otherwise be rejected as the work of a madman if the first psychiatric diagnosis were to stand.

The public outcry against the first report, together with the professional criticisms of the report's methods and conclusions, were sufficient for the court to request a second psychiatric report, which was published just one week before the trial began in April 2012. This report was led by two Norwegian forensic psychiatrists Agnar Aspaas and Terje Tornissen, who from previous criminal cases in which they had been involved both had a reputation of being less likely to give psychiatric diagnoses (Orange, 2012). Aspaas and Tornissen's assessment included the commissioning of a team of 17 experts who observed Breivik in Ila Prison 24 hours a day for 21 days, because the medical staff in the prison had also questioned the diagnosis of paranoid schizophrenia. The second psychiatric report rejected the Husby and Sorheim diagnosis of paranoid schizophrenia, and recommended that Breivik be judged criminally responsible for his actions, although it stated that he did suffer from antisocial (dissocial) and narcissistic personality disorders. In questioning the conclusions from the first psychiatric report, Aspaas and Tornissen argued that the so-called neologisms such as "national Darwinists" and "cultural Marxists" were perfectly understandable phrases, that many extreme far-right political groups shared Breivik's views about "Eurabia" and the like, that he had trained himself specifically to remain unemotional and to distance himself from the fate of his victims, and that his actions had been planned and carried out too carefully for someone suffering from schizophrenia (as Torgersen and Rosenqvist had previously suggested when the first report was leaked).

At the beginning of Breivik's trial on April 16, 2012, the court therefore had two conflicting psychiatric reports to consider, with further conflicting expert witness testimony to be added during the trial that extended the range of proposed diagnoses for Breivik to include Asperger's and Tourette's syndromes. One interesting feature of the trial is that the two authors of the first psychiatric report, Husby and Sorrheim, sat throughout the whole proceedings that lasted for over 2 months until its conclusion on June 22, 2012. Despite the opposing second psychiatric report and the weight of public and other expert opinion against them, Husby and Sorrheim stood by their initial diagnosis of paranoid schizophrenia. An interesting further observation made by Husby about the trial was that he observed that Breivik seemed to be aroused by the violence he had committed, and by his fantasies of killing even more people and of beheading Gro Harlem Brundtland. When questioned along these lines, Breivik strongly rejected Husby's observations and interpretation, though the links to the childhood report on his sexualized and aggressive problematic relationship with his mother do provide scope for further exploration. Unfortunately, however, the use of this early childhood report during the trial was blocked by Breivik's mother. On August 24, 2012 the team of five judges who had presided over Breivik's trial declared that he was "legally sane," that many extremists shared his conspiracy views on Eurabia, Islamophobia, and ethnic cleansing, and that he should receive 21 years in "preventive detention" in Ila Prison.

One of the reasons for presenting this detailed account of Anders Breivik is to emphasize the problems that even highly expert clinicians under the most exacting circumstances have in reaching an agreed diagnosis in such cases. Surely, the problems of diagnosis cannot simply be blamed on the knowledge or expertise of the respected clinicians involved; instead they are more likely to be a consequence of the fundamental flaws in the diagnostic systems themselves that lead to such high-profile contradictions. The suggestion that we will examine briefly here, but will expand in subsequent chapters, is the problem for the diagnostic and classification systems that we mentioned earlier—namely, "where are all the anger disorders?" That is, although the other basic emotions of anxiety, sadness, and disgust provide the basis of many of the existing clinical diagnoses (see Chapter 3), the lack of inclusion of anger and anger-based disorders, particularly in relation to violence, torture, rape, and murder, is really quite bizarre, so it must reflect a problem, we will suggest, with how society views anger, aggression, and associated acts of violence. The history of human violence, and its acceptance within our cultures, seems to have blinded us to its pathology in the form of acts of rape, violence, torture, murder, and, in its most extreme, in the almost constant wars and acts of genocide throughout our appallingly violent history. Of course, we must be grateful for some apparent improvement in our proclivity to violence as Steven Pinker has summarized in his thought-provoking work *The Better Angels of our Nature: The Decline of Violence in History and its Causes* (Pinker, 2011). However, our cultural acceptance of violence seems to have left it largely excluded from the diagnostic systems.

The Australian psychiatrist Paul Mullen pointed to something related to this argument in comments he made in an interview with ABC News Australia about Breivik and other individuals who have carried out such spree killings (see <http://www.abc. net.au/news/2012-07-22/forensic-psych-on-violent-minds/4146324>, accessed May 21, 2013). Mullen drew a comparison with the so-called culture-bound diagnostic category "amok," which is listed in the DSM as a type of dissociative episode. It was originally diagnosed in Malaysian men and comes from the Malay word meaning "mad with uncontrollable rage" and has now given us the phrase in English "running amok." The Malay believe that an evil tiger enters the (usually) young man's body and causes him to run wild and act aggressively toward others, typically in a crowded place, including attacking strangers with a sword or dagger. The outcome was typically that the amok person was either killed by those around him or ended up committing suicide after the killing spree. Those few who survived usually reported amnesia for the episode, hence its classification as a dissociative episode in DSM. It has also been likened to the Viking berserkers, who during battle fought with a wild trance-like fury, possibly induced by psychoactive drugs derived from plants and mushrooms, and which has given us the English word "berserk." Paul Mullen has suggested that the supposedly Malay culture-bound syndrome of amok over recent decades has now become part of a Western cultural script, in which typically a young isolated man who is obsessional and rigid in nature, and who has a fascination with things military, dies in a "blaze of glory" while killing as many other people as possible in the process.

The fact that DSM refers to amok as a *dissociative disorder* again misses the possibility, to be detailed in subsequent chapters, that it is an anger disorder in which the person typically regains honor and glory following a period of isolation, lack of recognition, and resentment against the world. These beliefs fuel a wild aggression, which helps the young man to overcome feelings of insignificance and inferiority, and to die a hero rather than a coward. Again, anthropologically, Rosaldo (1980) described the use of head-hunting by the Ilongot of the Philippines; this was typically carried out by young men in a state of grief as a way of using anger and head-hunting to overcome their unwanted feelings of loss and weakness. As a tail note to our discussion of Anders Breivik, it is interesting that unlike most of the previous spree killers he did not turn his guns on himself and commit suicide. However, when he eventually surrendered to the Norwegian SWAT team he is reported to have said to them that he was ready to die and that they could execute him on the spot, perhaps so that he would be remembered as a martyr rather than a suicide (Orange, 2012).

The Case Formulation Approach

The case formulation approach is sometimes presented as an alternative to the psychiatric diagnostic approach, especially in clinical psychology and psychotherapy, which is why we have chosen to provide a brief outline of it here. The formulation provides a possible model or theory about an individual's psychological problems in relation to key points in their history, likely causes and precipitants of the problems, maintenance factors that perpetuate the problems, plus some summary of additional vulnerability and resilience factors, but all of this account is framed in terms of a particular theoretical approach (see the excellent *Handbook of Psychotherapy Case Formulation* by Tracy Eells, 1997). A psychoanalytic formulation therefore would highlight the impact of early relationships on current unconscious processes; a cognitive therapy formulation would highlight the role of dysfunctional schemas, negative thoughts, and logical errors of thinking; and a behavioral formulation would highlight learning history and current environmental contingencies. Within each theoretical framework, key features of the individual's history and experience would be highlighted that offered proof of the framework's proposed model of how and why that individual developed those particular problems. The framework would also offer a set of goals for therapeutic intervention that would be likely to lead to some resolution of the psychological difficulties.

An example of a case formulation is presented here, taken from a more detailed case account that has been published previously (Power, 2010). Anna was a 30-year old newly married woman who had been referred by her GP because of her bulimia. Although she had developed bulimia in her early 20s, she had never previously sought help. She had recently discussed the bulimia with her GP because she was several months pregnant and was worried about what effect the bulimia might have on her baby. Within the emotion-focused cognitive therapy (EFCT) framework (Power, 2010), key elements from Anna's history and current problems included:

1. Anna's parents had an especially conflictual relationship, with her mother, the dominant one in the family, believing that she had married beneath herself. Her father had responded to his wife's dominance in a passive–aggressive fashion and had eventually developed an alcohol problem and had long periods when he left home, though he always returned. Because her mother needed to work, the maternal grandmother moved into the home, but she had been physically abusive toward Anna and her siblings.

2. Anna was lonely and isolated throughout her childhood and adolescence, on the one hand believing that she was too good for the other children but having considerable self-ambivalence because she also felt fat and unattractive as an adolescent. She was jealous of her older sister who was slim and attractive. She responded to these problems by working hard at school, which helped her to bury her feelings.

3. At teacher training college she met her current husband, though they had separated previously and it had not been an easy relationship because she felt

that he wasn't sufficiently interested in her. However, she did not talk to any-one about her relationship problems because that would be a "betrayal" of the relationship.

4. Throughout her teens Anna had at times used restrictive dieting in order to control her weight and in an attempt to be slim and more attractive. However, she had discovered that her slim, attractive older sister used vomiting and pur-ging after "overindulging," then tried it herself after a serious argument with her boyfriend, and found that it worked for her.

5. In EFCT terms, Anna was an emotionally closed person who had learned that emotions, especially anger, were extremely destructive in relationships and were therefore best hidden away. Her bulimia thereby served several functions, which helped to maintain or perpetuate the bulimia, including ridding herself of unwanted emotions while helping her to feel slimmer and more attractive despite the emotion- and interpersonal-driven binges.

6. One of the goals of therapy was therefore to help Anna learn to express emo-tions such as anger in a constructive way in her main relationships, rather than using bingeing and purging to rid herself of such feelings.

An obvious criticism of this brief example of a case formulation is that rather than offering an alternative to the diagnostic approach that has been discussed throughout this chapter it actually takes the diagnosis of bulimia as its starting point. So how could authors see the case formulation approach as in any way counter to the diag-nostic approach? One answer from people such as Pilgrim (e.g., Pilgrim, 2009) is that the "diagnosis" is not really a diagnosis, but just a shorthand way of referring to a set of behaviors or problems that in the case of "bulimia" include bingeing, purging, and vomiting. However, it is possible to see such a response as somewhat disingenuous in that the diagnostician might justifiably reply that the case formulation approach thereby includes at least an *implicit* diagnostic category or folk psychology category when terms such as "anxiety," "depression," "delusion," or "bulimia" are used, even if the psychotherapist only intends these as a "shorthand" for a more detailed descrip-tion of the problems.

In summary, therefore, although the case formulation approach is presented in clinical psychology and psychotherapy as an alternative to the psychiatric diagnostic approach, a fair criticism of such claims seems to be that at minimum *implicit* diag-nostic categories are used within the approach. Even worse, when case formulation uses terms such as "anxiety" or "depression," it is surely completely contradictory to use these terms while denying that they might have any diagnostic implications whatsoever. Although the case formulation and diagnostic approaches are presented as alternatives or opposites, in fact they are very much bedfellows in that case formulation at minimum uses implicit diagnostic categories about which it needs to come clean.

In the context of the case formulation approach, we will also mention the WHO International Classification of Functioning, Disability and Health (ICF) (World Health Organization, 2001) approach. Mike Berger (2008) has proposed that the WHO ICF approach could be an alternative to the existing diagnostic and classification systems. However, the ICF has a similar relationship to classification and diagnosis as the case formulation approach. That is, the ICF does not provide an alternative to diagnosis but rather spells out a range of personal and environmental factors that can impact on a possible diagnosis that then determines the level of functioning of the individual with the diagnosis. The use of an environmental aid could in fact lead the individual to have a superior level of functioning than average because the environmental aid provides a perfect correction for a disorder. Therefore the level of functioning within the ICF system is determined by an interaction of a disorder with a range of personal and environmental factors. The ICF system builds on, but does not replace, the diagnostic and classification systems.

Summary and Conclusions

In this chapter we have tried to offer a critique of approaches to classification and diagnosis in psychiatry. The current systems are predominantly the APA's DSM and the WHO's ICD. The two systems can be criticized from a number of perspectives. First, in contrast to the invaluable classification systems in chemistry and biology, psychiatric classification systems are deliberately *atheoretical*. As we have summarized, atheoretical approaches to classification in which categories are defined by consensus (or otherwise) of groups of experts are vulnerable to fashions and trends and the self-serving biases of the dominant members of such committees. Every few years therefore one watches as diagnoses such as homosexuality come and go as cultural and other changes impact on the expert committees.

One reaction to psychiatric diagnosis is therefore to reject it altogether, with particular diagnostic categories such as schizophrenia having suffered an onslaught from some in psychiatry and many in clinical psychology and elsewhere. We briefly considered the case formulation approach, which many in clinical psychology and psychotherapy see as a rejection of and an alternative to psychiatric diagnosis. However, the case formulation approach, when it presents itself as a rejection of the diagnostic approach, is vulnerable to the accusation that it incorporates *implicit* or folk psychological diagnostic categories; thus, terms such as anxiety, depression, bulimia, delusions, and hallucinations are commonly used as part of the case formulation approach, but without any systematic attempt to explore their structural relation to each other or to offer an explicit account of their definition. Such approaches therefore appear to replace explicit diagnostic categories with implicit ones. We would also add a comment on those psychiatrists who would try to limit the term "madness" just to the more "severe" psychoses rather than also including the "neuroses" (to use the old money term). In fact, as one of the anonymous reviewers of this book argued, such a proposal would be the equivalent of restricting Mendeleev's periodic table to just the metals, for example. It would also do a disservice to the people that such psychiatrists sometimes dismiss as the "worried well," for it is sometimes the "worried well" who kill themselves because of their distress, or who spend lives in poverty, misery, and with an increased risk of a range of medical problems. In this book therefore we will note that the lay term "madness" should be mapped onto the whole range of psychological disorders, not just the psychoses.

The approach that we will try to take in the remainder of this book is to explore if it is possible to produce an explicit diagnostic and classification system that is based on current psychological theory. That is, we will explore if it is possible to produce a theoretically based classification and diagnostic system. Of course, such a venture may simply find itself at the end of a very long cul-de-sac, in which case we might at least have the benefit of knowing what direction future explorers should *not* take. However, our hope is that we may find the *El Camino*, the true path to diagnostic enlightenment, but that even if we do not complete the whole journey to our Santiago de Compostela, then at least we might have pointed the diagnostic pilgrims who follow behind us in the right direction.

3

THE CURRENT APPROACH

When I build castles in the air,
Methinks the time runs very fleet,
All my joys to this are folly,
Naught so sweet as melancholy

Robert Burton (1621)

Introduction

The purpose of this chapter will be to present some brief background information about cognitive science, then within this general approach to outline how the SPAARS model (schematic, propositional, analogical, and associative representational systems) that we have developed over a number of years (Power and Dalgleish, 1997, 2008; Power, 2010) can be further extended to provide the theoretical basis for a diagnostic system. The SPAARS model was developed initially to give an account of the generation and regulation of emotion, and it is proposed that this account can provide a good starting point for understanding the range of emotional disorders; it also offers new analyses and understandings of the relationship of these disorders to each other, as any good classification system should. However, as we discussed in Chapter 2, the range of diagnoses of psychological disorders in systems such as DSM goes well beyond the emotions alone and includes a diverse set of biological, personality, and cognitive systems that, while they have some overlap with the emotion system, must also be considered in addition to it. The proposal that we will examine here is that the SPAARS model can nevertheless still provide a basic starting point; however, we need to examine, for example, how the SPAARS analogical system can be extended to incorporate biological and drive-related factors, and how the associative and schematic model systems can be extended to take account of the range of the various cognitive systems. To give the punch line in advance, we will argue that drive-related, emotion-related, and cognition-related factors can be incorporated into an expanded SPAARS model in order to provide a theoretical basis for classification and diagnosis. The remainder of this chapter, therefore, will be used to provide a summary of such an expanded SPAARS model. Each of the subsequent chapters will then examine drive-related, emotion-related, and cognition-related disorders in more detail.

Cognition and Emotion—Some Brief Remarks

The pioneering work of researchers such as John Teasdale (1983) and Gordon Bower (1981) began to open the cognitive-behavioral world to the possibility that cognition and emotion, thinking and feeling, interact with each other; that sometimes feeling states make us more likely to think in a particular way and, as in early cognitive therapy, thinking can lead us to feel in a particular way. Figure 3.1 expresses these ideas in a very simple fashion: Beck's initial cognitive therapy model considered the linear causal chain shown in Figure 3.1(a) in which cognition causes emotion (e.g., Beck et al., 1979), but subsequent work suggested that cognition and emotion may interact with each other, rather than one taking causal priority over the other (as shown in Figure 3.1b). Gordon Bower (1981) demonstrated that if someone is in a sad mood they may be less likely to recall positive memories and more likely to think about negative ones. Although there have been problems in replicating some of these early studies (see Power and Dalgleish, 2008) that work was important because it suggested possibilities for the emotional disorders such as in depression and anxiety disorders. What if vulnerable individuals are sometimes unable to protect themselves against certain types of thoughts or thinking once they enter a particular emotion state, even though under other circumstances they can?

Let us take the example of attitude and attitudinal change from the area of social psychology as an important example (see Chaiken and Trope, 1999, for more details). The majority of liberal-minded individuals would like to think of themselves as being free from prejudice and that they support non-racist, non-sexist, and non-ageist views and policies. That is, their stated or *explicit* attitudes demonstrate what fair-minded individuals they are. However, the truth tends to be less straightforward and more complex; when it comes to measures of behavior,

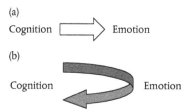

Fig. 3.1. (a) Cognition causes emotion. (b) The reciprocal relationship between cognition and emotion.

automatic perceptual processes, reaction time measures, and psychophysiology there may well be indicators of prejudice and bias that the individual would consciously reject (Chaiken and Trope, 1999). In other words, people's *implicit* attitudes may sometimes conflict with their explicit attitudes. A system that leads to conflicting attitudes occurring in parallel with each other cannot be readily accommodated in the cognitive therapy models that we have considered so far because those models do not allow for parallel, potentially conflicting, processes that thereby produce different conflicting outcomes.

There is of course a considerable history within other areas of psychology of the idea of potentially conflicting processes running in parallel with each other. Hermann von Helmholtz, the great nineteenth-century German scientist, had, long before Freud, argued for the need for unconscious or automatic processes in visual perception, and demonstrated conditions under which apparently integrated processes disintegrated or produced errors, such as in visual illusions (Power, 1997). The psychoanalytic approach developed by Freud includes preconscious, conscious, and unconscious systems which are typically in conflict with each other, and are often in conflict within themselves; thus, the unconscious system is not considered to hold information in a consistent and logical manner but contains contradictory and apparently illogical material (e.g., Freud, 1915). The model that we will present does not owe its allegiance to psychoanalysis but is squarely based on modern cognitive approaches to emotion. Our main point of departure from extant models in cognitive therapy is therefore in the need for two distinct sets of conscious and unconscious or automatic processes that sometimes act in a synergistic manner but at other times produce conflicting outputs.

In addition to the evidence for two such routes or sets of processes that we have briefly cited from the fields of social cognition and psychoanalysis, there is also increasing evidence from research in neuroscience for the existence of two separate routes. For example, Joseph LeDoux's (e.g., Le Doux, 1996) work on the acquisition and maintenance of fear in rats clearly shows the need for a fast fear-based system that operates through the amygdala in the mid-brain (i.e., what used to be known as the limbic system) and a higher route through the cortex. These two routes can operate in tandem and synergistically or can produce conflicting outputs depending on the exact conditions and circumstances. LeDoux's work with animals together with similar work in humans points to the need for more complex multilevel systems in order to understand emotional reactions in humans. Daniel Kahneman (2011) has also recently summarized a wide range of evidence that points to what he calls System 1 and System 2, which operate under different principles from each other but very directly map onto the automatic and conscious processing systems mentioned here. In the next section, therefore, we will outline our own SPAARS model of emotion and demonstrate the need for more complex models that do justice to the phenomena under consideration and provide a richer basis for the diagnostic and classificatory systems needed to work with a range of emotional and other disorders.

The SPAARS Approach

My colleague Tim Dalgleish and I have developed the SPAARS model over the past decade or so (Power and Dalgleish, 1997, 2008; Power, 2010). There have been a number of influential multilevel theories of emotion prior to our model, in particular the work of Howard Leventhal and Klaus Scherer (Leventhal and Scherer, 1987) and of John Teasdale and Phil Barnard (Barnard 1993) must be highlighted. We hope that we have incorporated only the best aspects of these models into our own SPAARS approach and left out some of the weaker ones.

The SPAARS model is presented in Figure 3.2. The first aspect of the model to emphasize is that we propose a number of different types of representation and processing systems, which are summarized as follows:

1. The analogical system. The analogical system refers to a collection of primarily sensory-specific systems that include vision, hearing, taste, smell, touch, and kinesthetic systems. These sensory systems provide the initial processing of external events that are usually emotion-provoking and for that reason often become directly incorporated into the perception and memory of emotional events. The system is also responsible for processing drive-related information from the internal and external environments, because when the organism is in a state of drive-related motivation both internal and external sensory systems are more likely to be deployed in the pursuit of and response to those drives. For example, in a state of hunger internal systems respond to bodily signals of hunger, while sensory systems are more likely to become vigilant for food-related stimuli. The combination of internal and external stimuli can lead to the generation of emotions within the emotion system, but an affectively toned state of hunger is likely to be produced that feeds into subsequent systems.

2. The associative system. This system typically operates automatically and outside awareness. It includes the innate-based starting points for the emotion system and other systems that develop over time according to associative learning mechanisms. Skills-based actions and repeated sequences also increase in

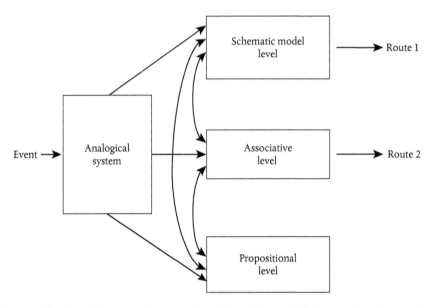

Fig. 3.2. The SPAARS approach to emotion. Adapted from Mick Power, Cognitive psycho-pathology: The role of emotion, *Análise Psicológica*, **27**(2), Figure 4 © 2009 Instituto Superior de Psicologia Aplicada, with permission.

their automaticity and become represented at this level, such that frequently repeated appraisal–emotion sequences can eventually occur automatically and outside awareness. Such automaticity often applies to drive-related sequences, for example in relation to food and sex, and according to socialization practices or traumatic experiences that can involve such drives.

3. The propositional system. This system is the one beloved of cognitive therapy in which verbal–linguistic statements (propositions) are represented. However, in contrast to cognitive therapy we do not believe that propositions directly cause emotions, but propositions such as negative automatic thoughts must be further processed either through the associative system or through the sche-matic model system in order to generate emotion. Nevertheless, the system may produce highly emotive propositions that are relevant to a person's men-tal state, such as "I am mad," "I am out of control," "I should kill myself," and so on, which, if subsequently processed in particular ways can be disastrous for the individual. For example, David Clark's well-known panic model (Clark, 1986) includes catastrophic misinterpretations of bodily sensations with prop-ositional statements such as "I am having a heart attack," "I am going to suffo-cate," or "I am losing my mind"; when such propositions are evaluated as true,

a vicious cycle is considered to ensue which both generates and maintains the panic attack.

4. The schematic model system. This is the high-level system in which dynamic and ever-changing models of the self and the world are constructed and which provides overall executive control. In relation to emotion, effortful appraisal of events and situations leads to schematic models that generate emotions; appraisals typically evaluate events and situations in relation to key goals, both personal and interpersonal, with the appraisal outcomes generating different emotions. The high-level dynamic models are especially important in madness; thus, if I believe that an auditory hallucination is the voice of god telling me to kill prostitutes (as in the case of Peter Sutcliffe, the notorious serial killer known as the Yorkshire Ripper), I am more likely to obey such commands than if I believe that I am suffering from auditory hallucinations which get worse when I am anxious but which I am now learning to manage. In both cases the initial experience may be the same—that of an auditory hallucination—but the evaluation of the hallucination is extremely different and has very different consequences.

These four proposed systems combine to produce two routes to emotion, as illustrated in Figure 3.2. There is a high-level effortful appraisal-based route that operates through the schematic model system and there is a low-level automatic route that occurs through the associative system. The operation of the two systems can be observed under many different circumstances and for many different emotions. A very simple example is the stepping-into-the-road reaction, when a fleeting movement out of the corner of your eye causes you to make a sudden jump back as you orient toward whatever was apparently moving toward you; further slower attentional processing via the schematic model system confirms that indeed it was a bus moving rapidly toward you and the feeling of panic increases because of the near miss. Alternatively, full attentional processing reveals that it was just a leaf blowing in the wind so you laugh it off and make a joke about it to your companion. This simple example illustrates one of the functions of the automatic associative system—the immediate interruption of current activity when the organism may have come under a sudden and unexpected threat that the slower schematic model system can then process in a more detailed and elaborative way, so that emotion and action become synergistic.

Later chapters in this book will of course be replete with examples of how the two routes can be in conflict with each other, but it is still useful to illustrate the point at this stage with a relatively common and persuasive example. Individuals who suffer from simple phobias (see Chapter 5) often report conflicting experiences about the phobic object, as in the following example:

> Jane was a nurse who had worked in hospitals all her adult life, but her job was just about to change and she was being moved into the community. She was referred for help because she was on the verge of giving up her career as she was terrified that she would come across dogs during her rounds and when making visits to people's homes if they kept dogs. She had experienced a phobia of dogs from a very young age, as had her mother, though on assessment she was unable to recall any traumatic or other negative experiences with dogs. In fact, when she thought carefully about dogs, she understood that people could be very fond of them and even have dogs as their best friends. The problem, however, was that she began to panic if ever she saw a dog, especially if one unexpectedly ran toward her or jumped up at her.

Jane's mixed reaction is not uncommon among people with simple animal phobias: on the one hand she reacted with panic if ever a dog was near her (i.e., emotion generated automatically via the associative route), but when she thought carefully about dogs she could feel mildly positive about them and certainly understand other people's positive reactions to dogs (i.e., an effortful appraisal occurring via the schematic model route leading to a mildly positive reaction). Many individuals with animal and other simple phobias often report that they know that their fears are "irrational" (a schematic model appraisal) but they are completely unable to do anything about their fear or panic because it is automatically generated via associative route mechanisms. Such fears and phobias provide dramatic examples of how the two routes to emotion generation can provide different and even conflicting outcomes ("I love you, but I also hate you!"). But we will leave further discussion of such examples to later chapters in the book when we expand on how these two routes relate to classification and diagnosis.

What is an Emotion?

So far in this chapter we have assumed that terms such as emotion and drive are understood, but in order to set the scene for the rest of this chapter in which we ask "What Is An Emotion?" and, later, "What Is A Drive?," we will start with an attempted, if lengthy, definition of emotion, which we have presented previously (Power, 2010). At least some aspects of the definition are controversial, but these are issues that will be picked up and dealt with in more detail in subsequent sections of this chapter:

> Emotions are mental and bodily states that typically comprise a constellation of physiological, behavioural, and psychological processes that follow the appraisal

or evaluation of a situation or event as relevant to the individual's goals. These goals range from basic drive-based survival goals to higher order interpersonal and aesthetic goals. There are a limited set of such emotion states that include fear, sadness, anger disgust, and happiness all of which have come to signal in a multi-task multi-level system shifts in the priority of goal-based functioning, and from which an infinite range of more complex emotions are derivable. These emotion states are normally short-lived in nature and need only last a matter of seconds or minutes; when they become more chronic they are normally referred to as "moods" for which the instigating situation or event may have been forgotten. The conscious aspect of an emotion is referred to as its "affect" or "feeling," though under many circumstances emotions can be unconscious and have no reportable affect state. (Power, 2010, pp. 18–19)

This definition of emotion offers a working approach that we believe will help to inform the clinical endeavors detailed throughout this book. However, it is worth noting at least some of the more controversial issues included in the definition, as follows:

1. The distinction between "mental" and "physical" states. This distinction is used here in a pragmatic way and does not imply any Cartesian mind–body dualism or split between body and mind. Indeed, the beauty of emotions is that they provide the integrating force between our own attempted splits between mind and body. However, these splits are not of the Cartesian philosophical variety but of a psychopathological kind that are more apparent in psychopathology and can become a necessary focus in therapy.
2. The concept of "appraisal." There have been many approaches to understanding the generation of emotions that can largely be traced back to the "feeling theories" of Plato and the functionalist theory of Aristotle espoused here. Functionalist theories have assumed that it is not events in themselves but how these events are evaluated according to personally relevant criteria that is important. Modern cognitive approaches to emotion, as we will show in detail later, are mostly appraisal based (Power and Dalgleish, 2008).
3. A goal-based definition. We believe that a crucial feature of events and situations is how they impact on our goals and plans and that different emotions result from different types of impact. As noted earlier, these goals include survival goals, interpersonal and shared goals, and aesthetic goals. Although emotions that arise from mnemonic processes might superficially appear to run counter to this goal-based approach, the content of the memory is normally about something that impacted on relevant goals and plans in the past. Similarly, emotions that arise from imaginative processes ("they would miss me if I

wasn't here!") typically involve events that would have an impact on goals and plans if they occurred in the future.

4. The proposal for "basic emotions." In the next section in this chapter we will examine some of the arguments for and against basic categorical approaches to emotion. Our overall view (Power and Dalgleish, 2008) is that there are merits to both dimensional and categorical approaches and that maybe these are not in such opposition to each other as is sometimes presented; it is certainly a step forward that DSM has begun to consider how categorical and dimensional approaches can be combined (see Chapter 2). For example, we argue that the starting point for the associative system is a set of five basic emotions, while at the same time we acknowledge that conscious affect can be described along dimensions of positive–negative, pleasant–unpleasant, calm–aroused, or whatever. In a multilevel system such as SPAARS, different levels may operate on different principles. Perhaps what is more difficult to reconcile is, as we will see, exactly how many basic emotions there are given that previous commentators have failed to agree on this issue.

5. Conscious versus unconscious emotions. There is nothing like the notion of the unconscious to divide opinion! Despite working together for many years on emotion and the SPAARS approach, my colleague Tim Dalgleish and I have simply agreed to differ on the concept of "unconscious emotion," a topic that divides the whole community of emotion researchers fairly equally (see Ekman and Davidson, 1994). Researchers such as my colleague Tim argue that for emotion proper to occur there has to be a conscious experience of affect (though in the absence of conscious affect what it is instead I am not quite clear—perhaps it should be called a "motion," which is perhaps what is left, following their viewpoint, if you drop the "e" for "experience" from "emotion"). Interestingly, even Freud (e.g., Freud, 1915) argued that there has to be conscious affect for something to be labeled an emotion: "It is surely of the essence of an emotion that we should feel it, i.e., that it should enter consciousness. So for emotions, feelings and affects to be unconscious would be quite out of the question" (Freud 1915, p. 104). However, for myself, the SPAARS model requires that we call the outcome of the direct associative route to emotion "unconscious emotions," because the associative route can generate emotion without conscious awareness. There are numerous studies of psychophysiology, subliminal perception, and dissociative phenomena that demonstrate the existence of emotion-type effects without conscious awareness, and the most parsimonious approach seems to be to call such states emotions.

SPAARS and Basic Emotions

The basic emotions that have been widely agreed upon and included in most modern lists are the five shown in Table 3.1. Almost all commentators would agree that the emotions of anger, sadness, fear, disgust, and happiness are "basic" according to a range of criteria, though we have drawn the list from the seminal work of Oatley and Johnson-Laird (1987). Ekman (e.g., Ekman, 1999) has done most to summarize what the criteria of "basicness" are: these include the universality of the emotion, its association with specific signals (e.g., particular facial expressions), its presumed innateness, its early appearance during child development, its fast and automatic generation, and a typically fast pattern of recovery. These characteristics do of course begin to change during development with the pressures of culture and family that shape the regulation and expression of different emotions according to "display rules," including the more pathological developmental pathways that are of particular focus in this book. In addition, more complex emotions develop with time, some of which may be unique to a culture, but whose starting point is one of the basic emotions from which they are therefore derivable (e.g., Johnson-Laird and Oatley, 1989).

We have argued elsewhere (see Power and Dalgleish, 1997, 2008) that the essential defining aspect that differentiates one emotion from another is its core appraisal, and we have offered a set of core appraisals in Table 3.1. These core appraisals are based on a set of relevant goals and plans for the individual. Let us consider briefly each of the five basic emotions. Each appraisal refers to a goal-based juncture, in which the goals are personally relevant whether in an immediate and direct manner or in a more indirect and abstract way. The five basic emotions will be discussed in detail in Chapter 6 when we consider disorders of emotions, so they will just be summarized at this point.

Table 3.1: Five basic emotions.

Basic emotion	Appraisal
Sadness	Loss or failure (actual or possible) of valued role or goal
Happiness	Successful move toward or completion of a valued role or goal
Anger	Blocking or frustration of a role or goal through perceived agent
Fear	Physical or social threat to self or valued role or goal
Disgust	Elimination or distancing from person, object, or idea repulsive to the self, and to valued roles and goals

Sadness is a consequence of the appraisal that there is an actual loss, or a possible loss, of a valued role or goal; thus, losses of key significant others involve the loss of that relationship together with a whole range of subsidiary goals and plans that are entailed in key relationships.

In contrast to sadness, *happiness* refers to the appraisal of movement toward or completion of a valued role or goal. In this definition, we restrict "happiness" to brief states such as joy or elation rather than the state of "life satisfaction" or Aristotle's notion of *eudaimonea* to which the highly overworked English word "happiness" also refers (see Power, in press).

The third basic emotion that we consider is *anger*. The key appraisal that we and others have proposed for the generation of anger is the blocking of a goal, plan, or role through a perceived agent.

The fourth basic emotion is *fear* or *anxiety*. We use these two terms interchangeably, though some previous authors have tried to make subtle distinctions between them (see Power and Dalgleish, 2008). The primary level at which fear is generated is at the appraisal of *physical* threat to the physical body. Alternatively, in some situations it may be one's *social* self and valued work roles and goals are under threat.

The fifth and final basic emotion is that of *disgust*. The origins of disgust in reactions to food and bodily products has been commented on since at least the time of Darwin (Rozin and Fallon, 1987). While we acknowledge the importance of disgust in relation to food and food waste, we nevertheless prefer to consider the relevant appraisal in terms of a more general repulsion toward any object, person, or idea that is seen as distasteful to the self and to significant others.

The disgust-based reactions that are seen in some of the eating disorders in which both food or certain foodstuffs and aspects of body shape and size become repulsive seem to be relatively straightforward, and we will consider these disorders in detail in Chapter 4. Perhaps less obvious is the role we have suggested that disgust, in particular self-disgust, plays in depression and in some types of phobias, OCD, and PTSD. In all of these examples there is some aspect of the self or world that is seen as unwanted and contaminating; thus in OCD it may be things that are seen as dirty or contaminating, whereas in depression it is part of the self that becomes unwanted and loathsome and that the sufferer tries to get rid of. We will of course consider these examples in detail later (see Chapter 5).

In summary, we believe that these five basic emotions provide the building blocks for our emotional lives and therefore for the full range of emotional disorders that are encountered. Before we look at these disorders in more detail, however, it is necessary to consider two further aspects of this approach to emotion. First, the idea that all other emotions are derived from one or more basic emotions; and, second, the related proposal that emotions can become "coupled" with each other in ways that can be detrimental and form the basis of some of the emotional disorders.

Complex Emotions

One of the central tenets of the basic emotions approach is that all complex emotions are derived from the set of five basic emotions. These derivations can occur through additional cognitive elaboration of an emotion, through the blending of different emotions together, or through the process of coupling mentioned earlier. Examples of cognitive elaboration would include worry as an elaboration of fear in which there is rumination about the future, and guilt as a form of disgust that is directed toward an action carried out by the self. Examples of emotion blends include contempt and nostalgia; thus, contempt, although listed under anger, typically includes a proportion of disgust combined with anger directed toward the person or object of contempt. Similarly, nostalgia, although listed under happiness, also includes a portion of sadness directed toward the person or situation that is the object of the nostalgia. Again, we will consider these issues in more detail in Chapter 6 when we return to the question of emotions and their possible disorders.

Emotion Coupling

We opened this chapter with a wonderful quote from Robert Burton (1621), "naught so sweet as melancholy," a phrase that might sound like an oxymoron but which from the SPAARS perspective illustrates how emotions can become "coupled" with each other, even so-called positive and negative emotions, as in "sweet melancholy."

One of the proposals that we made in developing the SPAARS approach to emotion was that certain emotion modules might become "coupled" with each other in ways that might lead to psychopathology (Power and Dalgleish, 1997, 2008). There have been one or two related proposals in the psychopathology literature, such as in the influential idea of "fear of fear" (e.g., Goldstein and Chambless, 1978) and the similar concept of "depression about depression." The fear of fear idea is especially relevant for understanding how someone who has experienced an extremely aversive state such as a panic attack might go to considerable efforts to avoid such an experience in the future; that is, they might successfully avoid having a further panic attack through continued avoidance, but nevertheless still live in a state of anxiety. We believe that similar couplings occur not just within emotion categories, such as in these examples, but also between emotion categories and that these couplings are often linked to psychopathology, as shown in Table 3.2.

Table 3.2: Examples of coupled emotions.

Basic emotion	Coupled emotion	Emotional "disorder"
Fear	Disgust	Panic
		Phobias (1)
		OCD (1)
		GAD
		PTSD (1)
		PTSD (2)
Sadness	Anger	Pathological grief
	Disgust	Depression
Anger		Pathological anger
		Morbid jealousy
Happiness		Polyannaism/pathological optimism
		Hypomania/mania
		Love sickness
		De Clerambault's syndrome
Disgust	? Fear	Phobias (2)
	? Fear	OCD (2)
		Suicide
		Eating disorders etc.

OCD, obsessive–compulsive disorder; GAD, generalized anxiety disorder; PTSD, post-traumatic stress disorder.

Examples of coupled emotions shown in Table 3.2 include: happiness–anxiety and happiness–anger, sometimes seen in manic states; anxiety–disgust seen in some phobias, OCDs, and types of PTSD; sadness–disgust seen in depression; and sadness–anger seen in grief (see Power and Dalgleish, 2008). Each of the examples in any individual situation is more complex than merely consisting of coupling, as will be shown in case studies in later chapters. Nevertheless, these provide examples of different types of coupling mechanisms. For example, in PTSD the victim may evaluate his or her experience of anxiety in a rejecting self-disgusted fashion, which can happen to some male victims of assault who saw themselves as tough and invulnerable prior to the attack; their feelings of panic and anxiety are now appraised as weak and pathetic, leading to feelings of self-disgust as well as anxiety. In this PTSD example, the coupling is caused by the appraisal of one emotion as weak and unacceptable thereby leading to a second emotion. In depression self-disgust can be coupled directly to the feelings of sadness, especially in some men with depression, but more typically the feelings of self-disgust are directed at the self in addition to any specific emotions. For example, following the break-up of a love relationship a woman might feel sadness because of the loss and anxious about how she will survive alone, while at the same time despising herself for needing a relationship and not being completely self-sufficient. In such cases, the coupling may be both direct and indirect in that it is more the cause of the sadness (that of needing a relationship) than perhaps the sadness itself that becomes the focus of the self-disgust (Power and Tarsia, 2007). We will consider the evidence for emotion coupling in more detail in Chapter 6.

The Drive System

We started this chapter with a detailed examination of the emotion system, although logically it might be considered better to start with the drive system because of its more primitive origins. However, recent work in psychology has focused on and produced more detailed models of the emotion system than it has of the drive system. Consideration of the drive system used to be more prominent in the early to mid twentieth century, with the American focus on behavioral psychology. However, in the computer age drives seem to have been replaced with a greater interest in cognition than behavior, and subsequently in emotion because of its clearer links with cognition. This refocusing is understandable in many ways because the links between cognition and emotion are much closer and have been of more interest to cognitive scientists than the links between cognition and drives. Nevertheless, most disorders of drive systems are secondary consequences of cognition–emotion disorders, for example secondary anorexia which can occur in some severe depressions as a consequence of the depression. Even when disorders such as anorexia are primary, they still include cognitive and emotional factors. Thus, anorexia as a primary diagnosis typically includes a range of cognitive factors such as beliefs about the need for control of appetite and food intake, and emotion reactions such as disgust toward foodstuffs and toward the body (see Chapter 4).

So what are drives and how do they operate? In order to distinguish drives from emotions, we should note first that emotions result from evaluations or appraisals (either conscious or automatic) of events that are of relevance to the individual; i.e., at the core of an emotion there is a cognitive appraisal of an event (see Power and Dalgleish, 2008). By contrast, a drive is a basic survival need that covers a range of physiological homeostatic and reproductive functions, including food, drink, oxygen, excretion, body temperature, sleep, and sex. Earlier drive theorists such as Clark Hull (1943) would have referred to this list as primary drives, akin to our concept presented earlier of basic emotions that are universal and therefore present in everyone. In addition, Hull and other drive theorists pointed to a number of secondary drives, which, they argued, emerge from our learning histories and can include the need for money, social approval, recognition, and power. Drive theorists proposed that such secondary drives will develop in some individuals but not in all, according to their different learning histories.

Clark Hull (1943) and others went further in their attempts to integrate drive theory within behavioral learning models. Hull argued that learning occurs via drive reduction, with states like hunger and pain leading to a homeostatic disturbance which requires the organism to learn appropriate methods to reduce it. Hence, if eating certain foodstuffs leads to a reduction in the hunger drive the organism learns from that and those foodstuffs are more likely to be eaten in the future. Drive reduction was therefore the key for learning in Hull's system. However, critics of drive reduction theory have pointed out that people sometimes seek out or deliberately create homeostatic disturbances, and that many pleasure-seeking activities, such as going to the cinema, can be drive-increasing rather than drive-reducing and we may learn to enjoy such drive-increasing activities. Learning therefore does not only occur through drive reduction.

More recent theorists have shifted away from behavioral language, especially in relation to the so-called secondary drives, to consider these as social needs and motives. Perhaps one of the most elegant and influential of non-behavioral theories has been Abraham Maslow's (1954) hierarchy of needs represented in the form of a five-step pyramid with physiological needs (drives) at the bottom, then safety, then love and attachment, then self-esteem and achievement, and ultimately self-actualization at the top of the pyramid. Maslow's proposal was that we will only move on to higher needs such as those related to self-esteem and self-actualization if needs lower down the hierarchy are being met. Although both elegant and influential, Maslow's organization of needs as a hierarchy has not received a great deal of empirical support (e.g., Tay and Diener, 2011). For example, to give a somewhat random example, a Buddhist monk might deliberately maintain himself in a state of hunger and sexual deprivation because of a religious belief which states that control of such needs is the way to self-actualization, contrary to Maslow's proposals.

Developmental and social theorists have also come to emphasize social and attachment processes as basic innate drives, in disagreement with the view of the earlier drive theorists that social motives were secondary drives. Harry Harlow's (e.g., Harlow, 1959) classic laboratory work with infant rhesus monkeys demonstrated that they became attached not to the wire objects that fed them (which on simple behavioral reinforcement principles they should have become attached to) but instead to the "terrycloth mothers" that were closer in look and feel to their real mothers, even though the terrycloth mother did not provide them with any food. Around the same time, John Bowlby's (e.g., Bowlby, 1969) initial work on children in care homes simi-larly demonstrated that even though a child might be fed and kept safe and warm, his or her social attachment needs were not being met under these circumstances and a variety of problems could ensue as a result. Bowlby's highly influential work has led to considerable understanding of the innate drive for attachment in infants and how it can become disordered because of environmental adversities. Bowlby proposed three styles of attachment in infancy: avoidant, secure, and anxious/ambivalent, though a fourth style of disordered attachment has been added subsequently (Main and Solomon, 1986). Hazan and Shaver (1987) have proposed that these infant attach-ment styles manifest themselves in adulthood in the way that the adult attaches in a loving relationship. They proposed that children with secure infant attachments who are allowed to be both affectionate toward, and independent of, their mothers are likely to mature into secure adults who are able to engage in comfortable intimate relationships with trust and a healthy level of dependence on their partners. Children with anxious/ambivalent attachment relationships to their mothers have learned to be clinging and dependent, or fearful of being smothered, or both. Such children, Shaver and Hazan suggest, are likely to become anxious/ambivalent adults. They will fall in love easily, they will seek extremely high levels of closeness and intimacy, and they will be terrified that they will be abandoned. The love affairs they have are thus likely to be very short-lived. Finally, the avoidant child who has been abandoned early on in infancy is likely, it is suggested, to become an avoidant adult. He or she will be uncomfortable getting too close, will have a fear of intimacy, and will have difficulty depending on others. Shaver and Hazan (1988) have amassed considerable support in favor of this formulation and similar formulations have been proposed by other authors (e.g., Bartholomew, 1990).

We will of course be examining some of the consequences of disorders of attach-ment in later chapters, beginning in Chapter 5, but in this section we need to consider how the SPAARS model can be expanded to take account of the various physiological and social drives that have been outlined. The simplified model in Figure 3.3 shows that, just like the processing of an event that leads to an emotion considered earlier, an internal or external drive-related stimulus will be processed through the automatic associative system and the high-level schematic model system. The simplified model focuses on the schematic and associative systems because these are crucial in the gen-eration of goals and plans, but propositional-level representations may also be gener-ated, such as "I am hungry!" or "I need sex!," even though these are not shown in the diagram. So let us take the example of an internal hunger-related stimulus such as the feeling of an "empty stomach." Such a stimulus may lead to certain automatic-level responses such as enhanced processing of food-related stimuli in the environment,

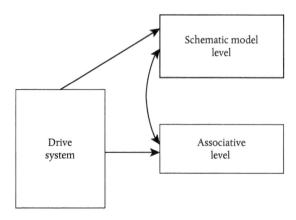

Fig. 3.3. Simplified SPAARS drive model.

which may be associated with an action tendency toward finding and ingesting food. However, high-level schematic processing might inhibit the automatic-level propensities, such as prioritizing a conflicting goal or plan along the lines of "I have to finish this lecture before I can go and eat." Alternatively, the schematic-level processing could be consistent with the associative-level propensity, so you take out your banana and start eating it while continuing with your lecture, to the amusement of your students. That is, the links shown between the schematic and associative levels in Figure 3.3 can be either facilitatory or inhibitory, as with emotion generation, depending on a variety of other factors such as the social circumstances. In fact, in addition to drive-related processes occurring through the different routes in SPAARS, it is possible that the one route such as the associative generates a drive-related action tendency, while another route such as the schematic generates an emotion about the drive. For example, in some types of sexual disorders (see Chapter 4) internal stimuli for sexual arousal could lead to a propensity for sexual action via automatic processes but come to be appraised as shameful via the high-level schematic model system and therefore be inhibited. Similarly, the acute onset of physical pain could lead to automatic processes such as quickly removing one's hand from a kettle that turned out to be hot, but then getting angry via the schematic system with the person who handed the kettle to you.

In this context we should make the general point that at least some drive states may increase the likelihood of certain emotion states, either because of overlaps between automatic systems at a physiological and psychological level or because the discomfort that can be caused by some drive states is likely to be appraised in a particular way by the emotion system. An interesting area of relevant research comes from Leonard

Berkowitz's (e.g., Berkowitz, 1999) work on his frustration–aggression model; in contrast to our own appraisal-based approach to emotion this has become an influential approach for the understanding of aggression. Berkowitz has argued that there are a number of drives or states that make people more aggressive. For example, Berkowitz and others have amassed a considerable body of evidence to show that anger, frustration, and aggression are much more likely to occur if people are too hot, in pain, thirsty, or in some other state of discomfort. However, as DiGiuseppe and Tafrate (2007) have recently argued, this body of data can also be taken as evidence for the automatic route to emotion generation within the SPAARS model. In a similar manner to how we can get angry with photocopiers and recalcitrant cupboards we can also get angry with states of our personal environment (too hot, too windy, or whatever) and states of our bodies (too hot, too sweaty, or whatever). There is no question that such reactions can occur without deliberate conscious appraisal via the automatic route, but even here these reactions are modifiable because of conscious appraisals. For example, if you have paid thousands of dollars to travel to a hot beach for your summer vacation, you are more likely to experience pleasure while feeling hot and sweaty lying on the beach rather than anger and frustration—the context and meaning of the situation is crucially important, not simply the temperature of the body.

A second point that we should consider is what is pain and how does it relate to drive and other states such as emotions? Simplistic models of pain might suggest that pain is the physiological response to the specialized pain receptors that occur throughout the body and pain occurs when these receptors are stimulated. However, we know from the work of Melzack and Wall (e.g., Wall, 1999) that there are important top-down influences (expectations, beliefs, etc.) on whether or not we experience pain at all even when pain receptors are stimulated. In this analysis, pain is a functional state which alerts us to the possibility of physical damage. However, if we reject the idea that pain is merely the label given to our experience of this physical damage then we need to replace it with something else. The standard functionalist line is that the physical damage activates a belief that we are in pain and it is the conscious awareness of this belief that gives pain its distinctive quality (Power and Dalgleish, 2008). So, there are two components here: the physical stimulus (activation of the pain receptors) and the activated belief. Under most circumstances, this belief will be due to the activation of the pain receptors by an event; for example the gash in your hand as the knife for the Sunday roast slips and cuts you rather than the meat. However, the fact that there are two components means that they can potentially operate separately and in some cases there will be no such activation of pain receptors but still an activated belief that you are in pain. This is psychogenic pain; here the experience of pain is an awareness of the belief that you are in pain even when there is no corresponding physiological event.

This approach leaves us with a concept of pain, drive, and emotion that is a combined awareness of both a physiological change and an associated appraisal, and a concept of pain (a sensation) that is an awareness of a belief that may or may not have been activated by actual physiological change. The fact that some form of cognitive evaluation or belief state is central to both sensation and emotion in this analysis means that any superficial consideration of the distinctions between emotions and non-emotions along the lines we have referred to above no longer holds any water. We can perhaps make some progress toward answering this question of the difference between sensations and emotions by reconsidering some of Descartes' ideas. As we have considered in detail elsewhere (Power and Dalgleish, 2008), Descartes drew distinctions between sensations such as pain and emotions such as fear by suggesting that the object that they referred to was in the body in the former case and in the soul in the latter case. In our discussion of this framework we pointed out that the notion of there being an object of emotions in the soul did not stand scrutiny. However, if we replace the idea of emotions having an object in the soul with the idea that emotions have an object that is cognitive we have the beginnings of a model in which we can tease apart sensations such as pain, drive states such as hunger, and emotions such as fear. That is, pain and drives may share their origin in a body state but emotions ultimately have a cognitive cause, the appraisal or evaluation of a relevant event.

Disorders of Drives

We have now outlined a range of biological and social drives, which together with the special response of pain we can consider in terms of whether or not there are possible psychological disorders associated with each of these systems. The main systems of temperature regulation, air regulation, eating, excretion, sleep, sexuality, and social drives will be briefly considered in turn; in addition we will also consider addictions such as gambling and substance abuse and somatoform disorders in general.

On initial consideration, breathing- and temperature-related systems seem to be exempt from being the core of such disorders, though, interestingly, asthma warrants careful thought because of the variety of factors that can impact on its development and course. In 2011, asthma was estimated to affect 235 million people worldwide and caused an estimated 250 000 deaths every year, mostly in low- and middle-income countries (see the WHO fact sheet on asthma, <http://www.who.int/mediacentre/factsheets/fs307/en/>; accessed June 5, 2013). The condition develops from an uncertain mix of genetic and environmental factors that cause chronic inflammation of the airways, including wheezing, coughing, and shortness of breath. A variety of things can exacerbate it, including air pollution, smoke, and allergies, but for many asthma sufferers intense emotions such as of anger or fear can also lead to an acute asthma attack. In fact, asthma sufferers have rates of anxiety and mood disorders that are two to three times higher than normal; the reasons for this are unclear though there are likely to be bidirectional effects between mood and asthma (Chatterji and Bergen, 2013). The point is that emotion and other psychological factors play important roles in the course and management of disorders such as asthma. Similarly, there are circulatory disorders such as Raynaud's disease in which the circulation and oxygen supply to the hands and feet can become severely restricted, resulting in extreme coldness and possible cyanosis. Again, extreme emotional distress can be one of the triggers for the acute onset of the disorder in sufferers. The point that we are trying to make here is not that we are proposing to include asthma and Reynaud's, for example, in our classification of psychological disorders but rather that disorders do occur in the basic air and temperature regulation systems in which psychological factors can play an important part. We will return later to the issue of somatoform disorders, in which similar biological and psychological interactions need to be considered, but first we will continue with our examination of the range of drive-related disorders.

Disorders of excretory function, or elimination disorders as they are referred to in DSM-5 (American Psychiatric Association, 2013), tend to occur in childhood and adolescence and include enuresis (problems with urination) and encopresis (problems with defecation). With both enuresis and encopresis there is a "primary" type in children who have never established any control over urination, and a "secondary" type in which the child has had a period of control over urination but then becomes incontinent again. As with many of the other drive-related disorders (see Chapter 4), there are often accompanying emotional and social issues that can contribute to the problem. The child may also become avoidant of certain situations and feel ashamed of their problems. The disorders tend to mostly disappear with development by late childhood or early adolescence, though in a very small proportion of cases they can persist into adulthood.

Food- and hunger-related disorders are everywhere around us and include anorexia nervosa, bulimia nervosa, and binge-eating disorder. Rarer disorders that are also included in DSM-5 (American Psychiatric Association, 2013) include pica, which is the persistent eating of non-food substances such as coal or metal, and rumination disorder, which is the repeated regurgitation of food. Emotional and social factors are significantly involved in the eating disorders, so they will be considered in detail in Chapter 4.

Sleep disorders are well known to occur in conjunction with a range of other psychological disorders, including depression, anxiety, substance misuse, and bipolar disorders. General problems with insomnia can include difficulty in initiating sleep, difficulty maintaining sleep, and early morning waking with an inability to get back to sleep. Other sleep-related disorders in DSM-5 (American Psychiatric Association, 2013) include hypersomnolence (excessive sleep), narcolepsy (lapsing into periods of sleep during the day), breathing-related sleep disorders (sleep apneas), and parasomnias such as sleepwalking and sleep terrors. Although nightmares are normally included as sleep disorders, their intensely emotional nature means that they should be considered among the emotional disorders, especially if they occur following traumatic events.

Sexual dysfunctions range from ejaculation and erectile disorders in men to anorgasmia and disorders of desire in women. The disorders can reflect a wide variety of influences that include medical conditions (e.g., diabetes and cardiovascular disorders can cause erectile dysfunction), cultural and religious factors, relationship issues, and emotional problems. Similar to eating disorders, therefore, the sexual disorders demonstrate the extent of interaction between all the different drive, emotion, cognitive, and social systems both for their normal and their dysfunctional operation.

The drives that we have labeled social drives reflect a complex of poorly understood factors that have become of particular interest in psychology and psychiatry in the past 50 years or so. We noted above the important work of Harry Harlow and John Bowlby in the 1950s onwards that highlighted the basic social drives for love and attachment in humans and other primates that could not simply be explained in terms of the behavioral reinforcement principles that were dominant at that time. More recent understanding of social development and of a range of neurodevelopmental disorders and their impact on social functioning highlights that our labeling of social relations as "social drives" is a considerable simplification of the factors that need to be coordinated in order to develop and maintain satisfactory competence in such relations. For example, poorly understood neurodevelopmental disorders such as autism may involve some unknown mix of genetic and other biological vulnerabilities in conjunction with social–environmental factors that impact in different ways on development, but which together produce a range of problems in social and linguistic communication skills and emotional functioning. Similarly, the quality of early caregiving, especially by the primary care-giver, will have a considerable impact, first with possible attachment problems and later with increased vulnerability to a range of psychological disorders, especially in conjunction with the experience of childhood abuse. Chapter 5 will be used to explore these disorders of social functioning.

We said earlier that we would also mention gambling and other addiction problems in the context of our discussion of disorders of drives, though again we must note the multiple influences and factors that can contribute to such disorders (see Chapters 4 and 6). We have included a reference to gambling here because the earlier drive theorists had labeled the need for money as a secondary drive, so if gambling is considered to be an excessive pursuit of money it could be conceptualized as a disordered drive. However, if, along with the substance-related addictions, the core of gambling is the pursuit of pleasure, excitement, or "highs," then gambling is better seen as an emotional disorder in which a range of extreme emotional states can be evoked in pursuit of the excitement and highs. We will therefore consider gambling and substance-related addictions in detail in Chapter 6.

The somatoform disorders as they were known in DSM-IV (American Psychiatric Association, 1994) have been relabeled in DSM-5 (American Psychiatric Association, 2013) as the "somatic symptom and related disorders" on the grounds that the term "somatoform disorders" was too confusing for primary-care physicians to understand. One of the main disorders, that of somatic symptom disorder, can include chronic pain in addition to excessive anxiety about one or more chronic physical symptoms that do not have a clear medical cause. These disorders span the pain, drive, emotion, and cognitive systems, but the importance of health anxiety or hypochondriasis means that we will consider these disorders under the emotional disorders category in Chapter 6 in addition to pain disorders in Chapter 4.

This brief outline of each of the fundamental biological and social drives has illustrated that any of them can become dysfunctional and disordered, sometimes to a life-endangering degree, and that a range of other social, emotional, and cognitive factors can impact on and contribute to such disorders in complex and often poorly understood ways. It is hoped that this brief overview of issues that will be dealt with in far greater detail in subsequent chapters has provided a sufficient grounding in the expanded SPAARS approach to classification and diagnosis, the basic principles of which I will summarize in the next section.

Classification and Diagnosis Revisited

This chapter has presented some detailed discussion of drives and emotions but has only considered the cognitive system in passing, namely how it impacts drives and emotions, in particular within the SPAARS model. However, rather than overload this chapter with an elaboration of the key cognitive systems such as perception, attention, memory, and executive functioning and how they may be involved in different psychological disorders, we will save this detailed discussion until Chapter 7. Of course, it must be noted that there are a number of neurodevelopmental and acquired neurocognitive disorders that affect the cognitive system, which will also be discussed in subsequent chapters including Chapter 7, but the primary focus of the present section is how the three systems of drives, emotions, and cognition can be used as a grounding for classification of the psychological disorders.

As a starting point, let us consider the way that symptoms are organized within the DSM in order to define syndromes or disorders. Table 3.3 gives the example of the key symptoms for "major depressive episode/disorder" that are specified in DSM-IV and DSM-V; it is required that five or more of the nine types of symptoms listed have been present for at least a 2-week period. However, when we examine these symptoms, and this is typical of all the DSM syndromes, the list includes a random mix of drive-related (e.g., appetite and sleep disturbance), emotion-related (depressed mood, guilt), and cognition-related (e.g., suicidality, worthlessness) symptoms. Symptom 7 in the table even manages to conflate the cognitive (feelings of worthlessness) and the emotional (guilt) categories, which are best separated because feelings of worthlessness are not inevitably accompanied by the emotion of guilt. The first step that is required with such a chaotic and random approach is to bring order to the system, which can be done as presented in Table 3.4, in which the symptoms are organized into whether they are primarily drive-related, emotion-related, or cognition-related. We acknowledge throughout that this tripartite distinction is primarily a pragmatic one, given, for example, the necessary overlap between the emotion and cognitive

Table 3.3: Main symptoms of depression from DSM-5.

	Symptom
1.	Depressed mood
2.	Anhedonia
3.	Weight change
4.	Sleep problems
5.	Psychomotor agitation or retardation
6.	Fatigue
7.	Feelings of guilt and worthlessness
8.	Poor concentration
9.	Suicidal ideation

Table 3.4: Symptoms of depression organized according to drive, emotion, and cognition.

	Drive	Emotion	Cognition
1.		Depressed mood	
2.			Anhedonia
3.	Weight change		
4.	Sleep problems		
5.	Psychomotor agitation or retardation		
6.	Fatigue		
7.		Feelings of guilt . . .	. . . and worthlessness
8.			Poor concentration
9.			Suicidal ideation

systems in that emotion generation typically involves cognitive appraisal processes. However, we hope to demonstrate the usefulness of the three-way distinction as a basis for classification of the psychological disorders.

Table 3.4 also incorporates a prioritization system: although we argue that each disorder will usually include a range of drive, emotion, and cognition symptoms, each disorder can also be specified as primarily a disorder of drive, a disorder of emotion, or a disorder of cognition, despite the involvement of the other systems in its presentation. In the case of the example of major depressive episode/disorder, the disorder is identified as primarily an emotion-system disorder with sadness as its focus, but it includes elements of the drive-related and cognition-related systems within it. Of course, as we will show in detail in Chapter 6, this description of depression as simply a sadness-related disorder of emotion would in this form fail to distinguish it from grief, which is also an intense sadness-related response (Power and Dalgleish, 2008). The crucial distinction between grief and depression is in the coupling of other emotions with sadness; thus, with depression sadness becomes coupled with self-disgust as a minimum, a coupling that is not present in grief (see Chapter 6 for a detailed analysis). It should also be noted that different basic emotions tend to have different characteristic impacts on drive systems. For example, in fear and anger the redirection of blood flow away from the abdomen and the non-striated smooth muscles toward the striated muscles in preparation for fight or flight is accompanied by a reduction in food- and hunger-based drives; similarly, feelings of disgust should reduce the sex drive, and so on. Different emotion states tend to have different biasing effects on cognitive systems, such as the narrowing of attention in anxiety, or the increased recall of negative autobiographical events in memory with depression (Power and Dalgleish, 2008). The three systems therefore tend to work in tandem, though they are likely to vary from person to person according to a range of learning and socialization experiences. One of the problems with a heterogeneous disorder like depression, as summarized in Table 3.3, is that different combinations of different coupled emotions can be seen in the various subtypes of depression, such that DSM does not know whether more sleep or less sleep or a decrease or increase in appetite are characteristic of the disorder because these apparently contradictory symptoms are likely to be the result of different emotion complexes, an issue that will be considered in more detail in Chapter 6.

The starting point for classification presented in Table 3.4 is therefore the identification of a *primary* drive, emotion, or cognition system together with what potential disordered forms of that primary system are likely to occur. It is inevitable that even though a primary system is identified as the core of a disorder other secondary systems may become involved, be they from the same type of system (e.g., drives with drives) or from the other two systems (e.g., drives with emotions, or cognition). One of the questions that arises with this approach is whether or not we have carved nature at the joints or whether each system has been randomly sliced and there are more appropriate divisions. Our response would be that the biological drives such as those based on food, thirst, air, evacuation, and sex seem reasonably straightforward, as we outlined earlier in this chapter. It is less clear what the precise social drives are and therefore which disorders are primarily based on social drives, though we will present the state of the art on this issue in Chapter 5. As we stated earlier, in recent decades the emotion system has been increasingly researched and laid bare such that the five basic emotions that we consider here and elsewhere (e.g., Power and Dalgleish, 2008) are generally agreed on by most emotion researchers. More complex, however, is the cognitive system and how best this might be analyzed. In fact we propose that two different types of analysis of the cognitive system are necessary in order to understand cognitive disorders and the contribution of the cognitive system to the drive-based and emotion-based disorders. The first analysis is along the lines of the traditional chapter headings from a book on cognitive psychology, which includes distinctions between perception, attention, memory, thinking and reasoning, and executive control. The second analysis cuts across these systems and looks at high-level typically conscious and controlled processes versus low-level typically automatic and unconscious processes that we have separated out in the SPAARS model; thus, each of the systems of perception, attention, memory, and so on reflect different synergies of conscious and automatic processes that can have important consequences for psychological disorders. For example, if somebody sitting alone in a room suddenly hears a voice talking to them such an experience will engage an interesting combination of automatic and controlled cognitive processes: perhaps non-verbal noises have been misinterpreted as verbal sounds; perhaps memories of familiar exchanges in that room with a recently deceased spouse have been recalled? In fact, the person in the room happens to be a psychologist who was drifting asleep and wakes up suddenly and says to himself "Oh, that was one of those hypnagogic hallucinations that you can get when you are drifting off to sleep." The consequences of the different high-level interpretations or schematic models of the same auditory experience are likely to be very different, according to whether the person (and others around him or her) labels their experience as psychotic, grief-related, or normal. Hence, the cognitive system is key to classification and diagnosis in two fundamentally different ways; one is the generation of experiences, in particular, at the analogue-associative automatic levels; and the second is in the high-level construction of schematic models of what those experiences are about. These schematic models are crucial for how we interpret or misinterpret all the different drive, emotion, and cognitive systems, as will be examined in subsequent chapters.

Summary and Conclusions

This chapter has covered a lot of ground, perhaps even too much, such that the reader has possibly been left a little bemused and even exhausted at the pace at which we have traversed the mountains, valleys, and lakes of classification and diagnosis. Along this marathon journey we have pointed to the importance of drives (both biological and social), emotions, and cognition and how these different systems need to be understood and related to each other in order to provide a necessary theoretical basis for developing a system of classification and diagnosis. We pointed to the SPAARS model, which, although initially developed as a model of emotion generation and regulation, can be extended to incorporate and understand the drive and cognitive systems. Indeed, the SPAARS model incorporates a multilevel approach in which conscious and automatic processes can operate in parallel with each other. We summarized the SPAARS approach to the five basic emotions of anxiety, sadness, anger, disgust, and happiness and then presented an overview of the different biological and social drives and how they may each become disordered. However, in order to classify and understand the psychological disorders we first need to specify for each disorder which of the primary systems (i.e., drive, emotion, or cognition) defines it, and secondly how the other two systems are also typically affected; that is, every psychological disorder will have a drive–emotion–cognition (DEC) profile in which the primary system is highlighted along with typical features from the two secondary systems. In the next chapter we will examine the biological drives and illustrate in more detail how this DEC analysis can be applied to a range of different drives and their characteristic disorders.

4

DISORDERS OF BIOLOGICAL DRIVES

Madness need not be all breakdown. It may also be break-through

R. D. Laing

Introduction

In this chapter the focus will be on the biological drives, which include food and related disorders, sexual disorders, sleep disorders, and somatic disorders. Because this is the most biological of the chapters, we will begin with some brief comments on the nature–nurture debate, which used to preoccupy biologists and psychologists but which in recent times has mostly been replaced by a more sophisticated question of which genes benefit most in which environments. That is, the question of gene–environment interactions, which we will deal with first in order to provide a developmental underpinning for understanding the origins of psychological disorders.

Gene–Environment Interactions

One of the perennial questions concerning the psychological disorders is that if, in evolutionary terms, they were simply disadvantageous to sufferers why have they not disappeared from the genome across evolutionary time instead of, as it would seem, actually remaining steady or even increasing? We will consider three possible explanations: first, that there is simple genetic inheritance but that a disease might not have its onset until after the main childbearing years; second, that there it is a chromosomal rather than genetic problem that reflects imperfections or vulnerabilities in the process of meiosis; and third, that the gene or genes might provide advantages under some environmental conditions even though they have disadvantages under others—these are the gene–environment interactions that are likely to predominate in psychological disorders.

There are a number of known genetic and chromosomal abnormalities that have profound effects on development, morbidity, and mortality. Huntington's disease is named after George Huntington, an American physician who in 1872 accurately described the disease and its inheritance pattern across several generations of a family in Long Island. This disease could provide a model for every psychiatric geneticist's dream in that there is a single autosomal dominant gene, the so-called huntingtin gene, which follows a simple Mendelian inheritance pattern. An affected parent will therefore have a 50% chance of having an affected offspring, but non-affected offspring are not carriers of the mutant gene and their children remain unaffected. Because the typical age of onset is in the 30s or 40s, prior to the recent possibility of genetic testing for the mutation many sufferers would already have had children before they knew whether or not they were going to develop the disease. When the disease does develop, there can be a variety of early presentations including psychiatric symptoms and mild cognitive problems that can appear before the characteristic jerky motor movements, which led to the earlier name for the disease, Huntington's chorea. These problems are the result of a faulty protein synthesis mechanism that damages cells in the brain and causes dementia, with a life expectancy of about 20 years after the onset of symptoms. The reason therefore for the continued presence of Huntington's disease is that disease onset occurs after most people with the mutation will have had children. Only now with modern genetic testing and genetic counseling is it likely that the disease will become less prevalent, because children and young adults at risk for having the mutant gene can now be tested before they decide to have children.

Down's syndrome is a chromosomal disorder named after the British physician John Langdon Down who accurately described it in 1866. In 1958 Jerome Lejeune, a French geneticist who made major contributions to the study of chromosomal abnormalities, identified that Down's syndrome is caused by an extra copy of chromosome 21, there being three rather than two copies (it is also known as trisomy 21). The extra chromosome copy typically results from a failure of disjunction of chromosome 21 during meiosis, so that two copies come from one parent, usually the mother, and a single copy from the other parent. The risk of trisomy increases with the age of the parents, especially with mothers and fathers in their 40s or older. The presence of the three chromosomes contributes to a variety of physical and psychological problems that emerge during development, including learning disabilities, delayed social and emotional development, distinct facial features, and increased risk of heart disease, auditory and visual problems, and early dementia. Together with the example of Huntington's disease, therefore, conditions such as Down's syndrome show very powerfully that problems with genes and chromosomes can lead to a whole array of psychiatric and psychological problems; that is, the presence of genetic and chromosomal abnormalities may be *sufficient* to cause psychiatric and psychological problems, but the perennial question is whether they are also *necessary* to cause such problems. We will return to this question throughout the book as we examine the range of drive-, emotion-, and cognition-related disorders. However, a more sophisticated approach has recently emerged in psychiatric genetics, which is the possibility that the same genetic starting point might be advantageous in some environments but disadvantageous in others, a starting point that is far more interesting than the previous simplistic nature versus nurture argument.

One of the classic examples in biology of a gene–environment interaction is that of sickle cell disease, in which a mutation in the hemoglobin gene leads to red blood cells that have an abnormal sickle shape. Although under normal environmental circumstances sickle cell disease leads to a considerably reduced life expectancy, in sub-Saharan Africa, where malaria is common, people with one copy of the mutated gene (sickle cell trait) have a survival advantage, with less severe malarial symptoms than people with two copies (who therefore have sickle cell disease). In areas of the world where malaria is rare, such as the USA, the disadvantages of the gene predominate and the gene is selected out through processes of natural selection, but in parts of Africa where malaria is still endemic (see World Health Organization, 2010) the advantages of the gene predominate so the occurrence of the gene has increased through natural selection.

Few things in psychiatry are of course based on the transmission of a single dominant or recessive gene, so there are unlikely to be any such dramatic examples of gene–environment interactions as with sickle cell disease. Nevertheless, researchers have begun to look for subtler versions of possible gene–environment interactions that might help us to understand both the possible advantages and disadvantages of predispositions that might lead to psychological disorders under certain conditions. Let us consider depression as an example. It has been clear for decades that there is a significant genetic predisposition to depression. Family studies show increased familial risk—the earlier the age of onset the higher the familial risk, and twin and adoption studies confirm a clear genetic component, though less for community samples or unipolar depression suggesting a smaller biological component (Hirschfield and Weissman, 2002). What is less clear is how this genetic risk translates into the expression of depressive disorder, because no evidence exists for true Mendelian inheritance. Family and twin studies also show that even the risk of severe life events may have a genetic component (Kendler and Shuman, 1997). That is, both the tendency to suffer adversity and to respond to it by becoming depressed can have genetic components. There are a number of theories about what could mediate such genetic risk. Suggestions include other biological changes (such as genetic polymorphisms), the risk of life events and responses to them, and other factors within the syndrome itself.

Several attempts have been made to look for polymorphic variation in gene alleles that might be linked to depression. This candidate gene approach initially identified a number of positive findings, but none have been replicated consistently. Recent genome-wide association studies, including a meta-analysis of 6000 cases, have not provided consistent findings (Wray et al., 2010). Rather than genes increasing the risk of depression in isolation, it is the tendency to become depressed in response to stressful life events that seems to be inherited. It is perhaps not surprising, therefore, that studies of gene–environment interactions have yielded more consistent results. These studies have begun to show that allelic polymorphisms of some candidate genes interact with life stressors to increase the risk of depression.

The first gene–environment study of depression focused on the 5-HTTLPR (serotonin transporter promoter-region) polymorphism and found that the short allele, associated with lower expression of the gene, was also associated with a higher risk of depression following stressful life events or childhood maltreatment (Caspi et al., 2003). In Caspi et al.'s study (the Dunedin Multidisciplinary Health and Development Study), over 1000 children have been followed up from birth to young adulthood. One of the key questions was why stressful life events lead to depression in some people but not in others. The researchers found that a short allele of the serotonin transporter gene was associated with greater response to stressful life events in comparison with those people with the long allele. Although this finding has been replicated in over 20 studies, some of the recent meta-analyses (e.g., Risch et al., 2009) have concluded that there is a lack of support for the original finding. However, it is possible that the recent meta-analyses have used a biased subset of the literature and an unreliable subjective measure of stress. The most recent meta-analysis, the largest undertaken thus far of 56 studies, has confirmed the association between 5-HTTLPR, stress, and the development of depression (Karg et al., 2011). In particular, stressful experiences in childhood have been shown to interact with the functional insertion/deletion polymorphism to predict the presence of depression (Karg et al., 2011). The childhood approach has also included investigations of resilience, with studies examining genetic differences that may constrain the stress response and increase the likelihood of resilience following maltreatment (Moffitt et al., 2005). So gene–environment models need to encompass both vulnerability and resilience constructs (McCrory et al., 2010). Very recent work on epigenetics has argued that the environment can actually shape genetic expression; thus, DNA methylation is an epigenetic event that affects cell function by altering gene expression. Future genetic research will undoubtedly investigate epigenetic modifications, such as DNA methylation, to the genome; this is a potential means of controlling the expression of genetic risk and may link an early adverse environment to later psychopathology.

Similar replicated gene–environment effects have been identified in studies of a gene encoding the corticotrophin-releasing hormone receptor 1 (CRHR1), which modulates the activity of the hypothalamo-pituitary-adrenal (HPA) axis, a system also thought to play a key role in the etiology of depression (see Power, 2013). Gene–environment effects have also been found for a polymorphism of the gene encoding brain-derived neurotrophic factor (BDNF), where the allele results in reduced expression of BDNF and confers increased risk for depression after childhood adversity; functionally, BDNF promotes neurogenesis in the hippocampus and may protect against glucocorticoid-induced reduction of neurogenesis (Juhascz et al., 2011).

One interesting question relates to the observation that depression tends to be recurrent, and that there is a tendency for each recurrence to be less dependent on precipitating stress, a process likened to kindling (see Power, 2013). Kendler and colleagues investigated the genetic contribution to this phenomenon in a large twin pair sample; they found that genetic risk tended to place people in a "pre-kindled" state rather than speeding up the process of kindling (Kendler et al., 2001).

This brief digression into modern psychiatric genetics has been presented in order to give a flavor of how at least some of our psychological disorders are likely to be the result of gene–environment interactions in which a genetic predisposition interacts with an adverse environment (whether biological, psychological, or social) to lead to disorder. The other even less explored side of this equation is the possible positive outcomes for these and other gene–environment interactions in which the polymorphisms may lead to *advantageous* rather than disadvantageous outcomes in order to help us understand their continued presence in the genome. Some of the work done by Jerome Kagan and others on child temperament and how it interacts with different types of parental caring styles to give different outcomes is relevant here, but this work will be considered in detail in Chapter 5 on social drives. For the remainder of this chapter, the disorders that can arise from the biological drives will be considered in detail.

Food and Related Disorders

Eating disorders often attract considerable public and media interest, with many magazines commonly discussing the difficulties of "celebrities" with their eating or their body size. Fairburn and Harrison (2003) point out that eating disorders are a significant source of physical and psychosocial morbidity, and they carry the highest mortality rate of any of the psychiatric disorders. DSM-5 (American Psychiatric

Association, 2013) groups eating disorders into three main types, anorexia nervosa, bulimia nervosa, and binge-eating disorder, with mention also of pica and rumination disorder (see Chapter 3). Our initial focus in this section will be on the three main eating disorders and how the relevant DEC combinations may distinguish them. However, we would note that obesity is excluded from DSM-5 and earlier versions of DSM on the grounds that a number of different factors (genetic, physiological, behavioral, and environmental) contribute to its occurrence. The logic of this exclusion is puzzling given that the same set of factors can contribute to other eating disorders such as anorexia. Therefore, for consistency we will consider both eating too much and eating too little as potentially dysfunctional even though various DEC profiles may need to be considered, as we will show. Across these main eating disorders are the extreme concerns about shape and weight, described by Russell (1970) as a "morbid fear of fatness." There is a tendency to evaluate self worth by body shape and weight, and an extreme preoccupation to be "thin," even in obesity where there may be repeated cycles of dieting followed by loss of restraint (e.g., Ogden, 2010).

Table 4.1 presents an initial summary of the disorders that can be associated with the basic drive of eating. There are variations in the basic drive that range from undereating, binge episodes in which there are periods of overeating, and consistent overeating. There is no assumption that across time someone only displays one of these dysfunctional types; instead people may shift between different patterns of dysfunctional eating behavior. The fact that some people shift between dysfunctional styles has been referred to as "diagnostic migration" and has led some experts such as Chris Fairburn and colleagues to propose "transdiagnostic" treatment approaches to the eating disorders in recognition of such changes (Fairburn et al., 2003). The crucial factor is that food and eating, for a variety of reasons, have come to be used in an

Table 4.1: Drive–emotion–cognition analysis of eating disorders.

Drive		Emotion	Cognition
		Disgust	Control
		Anger	Autonomy
	Under		
		Disgust	Self-comfort
Eating	Binge	Anger	Regulation
			Rejection
	Over		
		Anger	
		Sadness	Self-comfort
		Anxiety	

attempt to respond to and regulate a range of physiological and psychological factors such as the emotion and cognition summaries shown in Table 4.1.

Our analysis and understanding of the range of emotions associated with the different eating disorders is at a surprisingly early stage. Hilde Bruch (1973, 1978), in her classic psychoanalytic studies of eating disorders, pointed to the role of important socialization and accompanying emotion regulation factors in children who went on to develop eating disorders, work that is only now beginning to be followed up (e.g., Fox et al., 2012). There is a growing body of evidence that suggests there may be problems with attachment in the history of people with eating disorders, especially anorexia nervosa. Early relationships have been regarded as a cornerstone in helping the child to learn skills of affect regulation, and problems with these attachments may lead the child to develop alexithymia. According to Taylor et al. (1997), alexithymia includes a number of difficulties in the identification of feelings, in distinguishing feelings from bodily sensations of emotional arousal, and in the ability to describe feelings to other people. A number of research studies have identified a relationship between the symptomatology of eating disorders and alexithymia, in particular with anorexia nervosa (e.g., Schmidt et al., 1993).

The discussion of whether or not childhood abuse (sexual, physical, or emotional) plays an etiological role in eating pathology has attracted much attention in recent years. Some authors have argued that there does appear to be a connection between bulimic symptomatology and childhood sexual abuse (Smolak and Levine, 2007), while other authors have stated that the relationship between childhood sexual abuse and eating pathology is overstated (e.g., Polivy and Herman, 2002). These authors discussed how childhood sexual abuse is also associated with depression and other psychological disturbances, and hence specific effects cannot be concluded. Smolak and Levine (2007) argued that there is sufficient evidence to link bulimic symptoms with a history of childhood sexual abuse, though it is still not clear for anorexia-restricting symptoms. They also discussed how some evidence is beginning to suggest that other forms of trauma (both in childhood and in adulthood) may well be related to eating/body image disturbance. In considering the nature of the possible relationship between childhood abuse and psychopathology, Andrews (1995) found that body shame moderates the relationship between abusive experiences (both adult and child) and depression. In a follow-up study, Andrews (1997) demonstrated that the relationship between bulimic symptomatology and childhood abuse was moderated by bodily shame. The findings suggest that abuse may play a role in the development of bodily shame and any subsequent depression/eating pathology, though clearly there are many other routes into the eating disorders.

The small amount of recent research into which emotions may be problematic in the eating disorders has begun to highlight certain basic emotions. In a number of studies of anorexia and bulimia, John Fox and colleagues (see Fox et al., 2012, for a recent summary) have highlighted that the emotions of disgust, anger, and fear warrant particular attention. We have already noted the importance of shame in the work of Andrews (1997), which is analyzed within the SPAARS framework as a form of self-disgust. However, problems with anger expression can become coupled with disgust in eating disorders such as anorexia and bulimia (e.g., Fox et al., 2013); thus, disgust is ultimately an emotion whose action tendency is to rid the body of unwanted material. This process of elimination begins as a process of eliminating unwanted body products such as urine or feces, plus the rejection of unwanted foodstuffs, but through development and socialization it comes to encompass emotions themselves, such that unwanted emotions are eliminated, and it generalizes further to moral behavior and interpersonal relationships. The work of John Fox and others has begun to point to anger as a particularly problematic emotion for people with eating disorders, and the traditional preponderance of women and girls with anorexia and bulimia may be in part due to the genderization of the emotion of anger as a strong male emotion which women were traditionally not allowed to express (Power and Dalgleish, 2008).

Work needs to be done in relation to obesity to explore the range of emotions and cognitions that may be typical of both binge eating and overeating. However, we have some preliminary relevant evidence from studies of binge-eating episodes in bulimia. Initial cognitive-behavioral models of bingeing in bulimia identified a number of vicious cycles involving dieting, beliefs about the importance of body shape, and low self-esteem that serve to maintain a pattern of bingeing, but which in bulimia is normally followed by purging (e.g., Fairburn et al., 1986). These cognitive-behavioral approaches have begun to be supplemented with greater awareness of the role of emotion factors, for example the feeling of emotional distress being a trigger for some bingeing episodes (Fairburn, 1996), though negative mood states more generally seem to increase significantly the risk of bingeing (Hilbert and Tuschen-Caffier, 2007). Any short-term benefit from bingeing to rid oneself of negative affect is typically lost because of the feelings of guilt and shame the person may subsequently feel in response to the bingeing episodes, especially where the disorder leads to overweight or obesity problems. However, the majority of obese individuals do not have a binge-eating disorder, even if once in a while they do binge (DSM-5 requires a minimum of one binge-eating episode per week in order to diagnose binge-eating disorder). One thing that is clear from studies of people with obesity is that the "jolly, fat" stereotype may be something of a fantasy; thus, studies show that there are a significant proportion of obese people who experience recurrent negative affect which has become integrated into their patterns of eating (e.g., Jansen et al., 2008). Of course, there are many different factors that can contribute to obesity, the complexity of which has led the DSM to avoid listing obesity as a psychological disorder. Nevertheless, whatever combination of cultural factors, ease of access to food, genetic predispositions (especially gene–environment interactions of the type noted earlier), and socialization factors may contribute to a particular case of obesity, there is an alarming increase in the rate of this heterogeneous disorder in modern society that needs to be both understood and tackled. Identification of different subtypes of obesity according to different DEC combinations would certainly provide a worthwhile area for future research.

Elimination Disorders

Table 4.2 presents a DEC analysis for the related elimination disorders. Following a similar structure to that presented for the eating disorders, there should be both disorders of under-control and over-control. The disorders of under-control include primary enuresis and primary encopresis in which the child has failed to gain initial sphincter control, and secondary disorders in which control has been established but is then lost again. The disorders of over-control tend to be combined with under-control in DSM; for example DSM-5 includes the subtype of "Encopresis with constipation" in which the constipation can develop for psychological reasons including anxiety about defecating in public places, or oppositional behavior by children, the result of which can be overflow incontinence. However, it may be preferable to separate out the under-control and over-control disorders because the primary reasons for the problem of under-control and over-control are likely to be very different.

The problems of under-control are commonest in childhood in which the child fails to gain control over urination in enuresis or defecation in encopresis. Because control of elimination is a developmental task to be achieved by the child, DSM does not diagnose enuresis or encopresis until a minimum age of 4 or 5 years. DSM-5

Table 4.2: Drive–emotion–cognition analysis of elimination disorders.

Drive		Emotion	Cognition
Elimination →	Under	Anxiety Shame	Control
Elimination ↘	Over	Disgust Anxiety	Control

(American Psychiatric Association, 2013) reports the prevalence of enuresis to be 5–10% in 5-year-olds, declining to approximately 1% in those aged 15 or older, whereas encopresis affects only 1% of 5-year-olds though it is more frequent among boys than girls. Both enuresis and encopresis seem to be associated with inconsistent or problematic toilet training and psychosocial stress, though physiological factors may also contribute, especially if the child is in receipt of certain types of medication.

Problems of over-control can also result from problematic toilet training and psychosocial stress, though again something as simple as medication that causes constipation with painful defecation may lead the child to the avoidance of toileting and withholding in order to avoid pain. One of the classic descriptions of the withholding problem was Freud's description of the "anal-retentive type" (Freud, 1905), which is a child who, in Freudian developmental terms, is fixated at the anal stage of development. The anal stage of psychosexual development is, in Freud's approach, the second stage that follows the oral stage as the primary erogenous zone and occurs between approximately 1 and 3 years of age. One of the key tasks of this stage is learning to control toileting, but if toilet training by the parent is too harsh there is a risk that the child may develop personality traits that become fixated at this stage, with the "anal-retentive" type being stubborn, withholding, and miserly. Although there is little empirical evidence to support Freud's theories of development, concepts such as the anal-retentive type have nevertheless entered our everyday language and, if asked, most people can think of one or more people they are acquainted with who fit such a description. However, it is unlikely that such traits originated solely in toilet training.

One of the key points about these elimination disorders is that although they can arise for non-psychological reasons, such as in early childhood or in older adults following significant cognitive decline, even in these cases a range of emotion and cognitive factors may come to play important roles in maintaining the disorders. Similar to the eating disorders therefore there are clear cognitive issues around control and loss of control that are represented by elimination; indeed, the concept of elimination needs to be extended to include some of the additional elimination techniques that are prominent in eating disorders such as bulimia, in which purging through vomiting and/or laxative use is done to eliminate the unwanted foodstuff quickly from the body. There is an argument therefore that bulimia is in fact a combined eating–elimination disorder because of its characteristic combination of bingeing and voluntary purging. The key emotions around eating and elimination are initially disgust-based because part of the function of disgust is to protect the body from dangerous foodstuffs and then to eliminate potentially toxic waste products from the body (Power and Dalgleish, 2008). Indeed, the initial reaction of "distaste" can be observed in newborn infants if they are given lemon juice to taste, as shown in the study by

Rosenstein and Oster (1988) with 2-hour-old babies. However, the complexities of our socialization, religious, and familial practices around eating and elimination lead developmentally to a wide possible range of emotions and cognitions becoming additionally associated with eating and elimination, a few of which are summarized in Tables 4.1 and 4.2.

Irritable bowel syndrome (IBS) is an example of an elimination disorder in older children and adults that has no known organic cause. IBS involves significant changes in bowel habits such as excessive diarrhea, excessive constipation, or alternating periods between the two. A range of symptoms can occur in IBS including chronic pain, fatigue, feelings of bloating, urgency of bowel movements, headache, and backache. Estimates vary, but upwards of 60% of people with IBS also appear to have comorbid anxiety disorders or depression (e.g., Whitehead et al., 2002). A range of factors can precede the onset of the disorder, including gastrointestinal infection and psychosocial stress. A study by Kennedy et al. (2005) compared the effectiveness of CBT and the antispasmodic drug mebeverine in a randomized controlled trial. The CBT consisted of six sessions of face-to-face contact at weekly intervals, which adapted Lang's three-systems model such that links between cognitive, behavioral, and emotional or physiological responses were linked to show how changes in one system may cause a change in another (e.g., Lang, 1985), an approach that is very consistent with the current DEC analyses of disorders. The CBT included psychoeducation about the nature of IBS, behavioral techniques aimed at improving bowel habits, cognitive techniques to address unhelpful thoughts related to the syndrome, and techniques to reduce symptom focusing, manage stress, and prevent relapse. The study showed clear benefits on a range of measures, including psychosocial functioning, of the addition of CBT to the drug treatment, with reduction in anxiety perhaps being key to the CBT intervention. What such studies illustrate is the connectedness between physical and psychological functioning in which, for example, the possible coupling of the emotions of anxiety and disgust may lead to an elimination type disorder such as IBS, though such putative emotion mechanisms await initial research. Interestingly, de Jong et al. (2011) found that over 68% of a sample of 64 people with bulimia also suffered from IBS, highlighting the possibility of an important overlap between these two disorders, as we noted earlier when we suggested that bulimia is an eating–elimination type disorder.

An additional complexity for the elimination disorders is the proximity of the anus and the urethra to the genital areas in both men and women. A strange design indeed to build the pleasure zone in the sewage works. As we noted earlier, Freud (1905) in his theory of psychosexual development argued in fact that the erogenous zones shifted from the mouth, to the anus, to the genitals such that any fixations during psychosocial development could leave these areas as the primary erogenous zones. However, we will deal with the disorders of sexuality in the next section, while noting some of the possible overlap with the elimination disorders.

Sexual Disorders

A summary of the sexual disorders is presented in Table 4.3. Following our approach to the eating and elimination disorders in which we considered the extremes of under-activity and overactivity, a similar approach can be taken to the sexual disorders. Furthermore, as with many of the eating and elimination disorders, although the impact of the disorder is on the performance of the drive, because of learning, developmental, and social factors the "cause" of the disorder can be at the emotion and cognition level, which is where any interventions may need to be targeted. We should also note that whereas eating and elimination disorders may have immediate survival consequences for the individual, too much or too little sexual activity has no such obvious consequences for the individual. Indeed, in many species the processes of sexual selection mean that because of competition and status between adult members of the species some animals might not engage in any sexual activity whereas others engage in a considerable amount. As Richard Dawkins expresses it in *The Selfish Gene*:

> One of the most desirable qualities a male can have in the eyes of a female is . . . sexual attractiveness itself. A female who mates with a super-attractive he-man is more likely to have sons who are attractive to females of the next generation, and who will make lots of grandchildren for her (Dawkins, 2006, p. 158).

In some species, such processes of sexual selection have led to some extraordinary outcomes for the males. As Dawkins comments with the example of birds of paradise:

> Extravagances such as the tails of male birds of paradise may therefore have evolved by a kind of unstable, runaway process. In the early days, a slightly longer tail than usual may have been selected by females as a desirable quality in males, perhaps because it

Table 4.3: Drive–emotion–cognition analysis of sexual disorders.

Drive	Emotion	Cognition
Under	Anxiety	Inadequacy
	Shame	Impotence
Sex		
Over [+Inappropriate]	Aggression	Domination

betokened a fit and healthy constitution . . . Females followed a simple rule: look all the males over, and go for the one with the longest tail (Dawkins, 2006, p. 158).

We have digressed into the subject of sexual selection as a warning about the difficulty of defining "disorder," because sexual disorders highlight the questions of norms and values and how they can be erroneously used to define disorder. Thus, in Chapter 2 we reviewed the DSM problem with "homosexuality" and how it used to be defined as a disorder while the more recent editions of DSM no longer do so. Homosexuality could be defined as a "disorder" on the normative grounds that it is practiced only by a minority, or on the value grounds that, for example, it is not acceptable within certain religious doctrines. When the value approach is taken to defining disorder, as in a religious approach to homosexuality, the consequences of the "diagnosis" are more likely to be that the condition is illegal or sinful and thereby warrants punishment, in contrast to the psychiatric diagnostic approach which, at least in theory, should lead to treatment for the disorder rather than punishment (though as we saw in Chapter 1, many so-called psychiatric treatments down the centuries have been far worse than any punishments).

A further issue that arises with the problem of the definition of the sexual disorders is that the prime motive for some types of sexual activity may be as much about domination and expression of status as it is about sexual activity. For example, the alpha male in some groups of primates such as chimpanzees may mount and engage in sexual activity with younger and less dominant males who allow themselves to be mounted as a display of submissiveness and thereby avoid a dangerous fight with a stronger male (De Waal, 1996). Studies of sexuality in human prisoners illustrate similar phenomena to those observed in other primates. For example, Knowles (1999) reported that in same-sex prisons homosexual activity between male inmates is typically used to express dominance–subordinate relations, with most male rapes in US prisons being rapes of whites by blacks, with the interpretation that prison allows the reversal of dominance–subordinate relations that are experienced outside prison. Interestingly, within the prison system, the dominant male in such sexual activity is not considered to be homosexual whereas the subordinate is, on the grounds that a "real man" would not allow himself to be dominated sexually.

In terms of psychiatric disorders in humans, the expression of such domination in which there is forced rather than consensual sexual activity is classed under the "inappropriate" category in Table 4.3. Such inappropriate activities includes things such as rape in general and pedophilia, in both of which there is a perpetrator and a victim and force or other inappropriate means have been used to make the victim engage in the sexual activity. Moreover, the issue of domination as an aspect of such sexual activity arises because of the nature of the figures for crimes such as murder,

rape, and incest. Recent figures from the US Federal Bureau of Investigation (see
<http://www.fbi.gov/>) show that in only 7.6% of the 15 760 murders committed in
the USA in 2009 was the murderer female. If we look specifically at murder of marital
partners, 141 husbands were murdered by wives, but 609 wives were murdered by
husbands (a ratio of 4.3 to 1 for male to female murderers); similarly, 138 boyfriends
were murdered by girlfriends, but 472 girlfriends were murdered by boyfriends (a
ratio of 3.4 to 1 male to female murderers). Crimes of violence between intimate partners were 82 360 incidents for male victims, but 564 430 incidents for female victims
(a ratio of 6.9 to 1 for male to female perpetrators of violence), and in the case of sexual
assault and rape there were 55 110 female victims but no male victims. For the crime
of incest specifically, a variety of factors mean that the figures are notoriously unreliable and likely to be considerable underestimations; nevertheless, in 2011 Statistics
Canada published a national study called *Family Violence in Canada: A Statistical Profile*
(see <http://www.statcan.gc.ca/>). This study showed that, for children aged 0 to 15
years, 69% of the victims of sexual abuse were girls and 31% were boys. The perpetrators of sexual abuse were the biological mother in 3% of cases, a stepmother in 2%,
the biological father in 8%, and a stepfather in 8%. In 44% of cases the perpetrator was
an older male sibling, uncle, grandfather, or other relative. Overall, what these figures
for murder, violence, sexual assault, and incest dramatically illustrate is that men are
many times more likely to be the perpetrators of such crimes, whereas women are
many times more likely to be the victims. The majority of crimes, especially those
of a sexual nature, are carried out by men, not by women, and dominance has to be
considered as a significant contributing factor.

Having spent some time in consideration of the "inappropriate" categories of sexual activity and the interesting problems that they raise for the concept of "disorder,"
we can now return to the categories of disorders that may be related to underactivity
or overactivity and to see what further issues such "disorders" might raise in terms
of our understanding of the contribution of norms and values to the definition of
"disorder." If we consider the category of "underactivity," then such issues only usually become defined as problematic when they are experienced in a sexual relationship; thus, problems such as delayed ejaculation and erectile dysfunction in men,
anorgasmia and painful intercourse in women, and lack of sexual interest or desire
in both men and women may well be experienced as unproblematic if the person is
single, but become problematic once in a relationship. The couple may then come to
an adaptation or compromise around the problem, so that it is normalized within
the relationship, or the couple may seek professional help in which case the problem
becomes a diagnosis. The issue that these examples raise is equivalent to that in our
consideration in Chapter 3 of the biopsychosocial approach that is captured in the

WHO ICF (World Health Organization, 2001), which some authors some have suggested might form a more appropriate approach to "diagnosis" (e.g., Berger, 2008). The ICF uses as its framework the biopsychosocial model of disability that represents a synthesis of the medical and social models, rather than a mere adoption of one or the other. However, as we noted, the weakness at the core of the ICF is that it adopts the ICD diagnosis as its starting point, so contrary to what Berger (2008) has proposed, it is not an alternative to the DSM–ICD atheoretical systems. Nevertheless, the strength of the ICF is that it can be used to describe health and health-related states associated with every condition and thus has universal application. The domains contained in the ICF are described from the perspective of the body, the individual, and society in four basic components; namely, body functions, body structures, activities and participation, and contextual factors, as shown in Figure 4.1.

The contextual factors are divided into environmental factors that make up the physical, social, and attitudinal environment in which people live and conduct their lives and personal factors, which include aspects of personality that may offer resilience or vulnerability to certain disorders. These factors can have a positive or negative influence, facilitating or hindering an impact on an individual's health and functioning. For example, a major factor influencing health is nutrition. Unhealthy diets, insufficient or excessive intakes of certain nutrients, may lead to cardiovascular diseases, diseases of the digestive system, metabolic disorders, and deterioration of quality of life. The main aim of a recent study that we carried out was to introduce

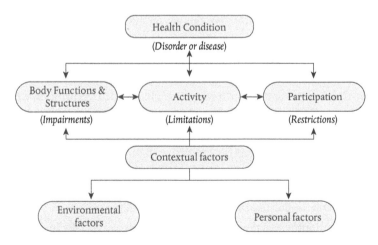

Fig. 4.1. The World Health Organization ICF model. Reproduced with permission from ICF Practical Manual, page 7, box 1 <http://www.who.int/classifications/icf/en/> © 2001, World Health Organization Press.

the Health and Functioning ICF-60 (HF-ICF-60), a measure of health and functioning that drew directly from the ICF and included the following domains: body functions; activities and participation; environmental factors (individual environment and social environment; Tutelyan et al., 2014). The chapters that cover body structures in the ICF were therefore not included. It is important to note that the measure builds on other international exercises such as the ICF-based development of the WHO's Disability Assessment Schedule, the WHODAS 2.0, which includes the six domains of cognition, mobility, self-care, getting along, life activities, and participation. A simple example of the management of a health condition that may lead to no disability is that of myopia or short-sightedness. Myopia could cause significant impairment, but it is now mostly overcome using contact lenses or glasses, which thereby provide a facilitative or assistive environmental factor such that aided visual functioning may be better than the normative level with the assistive factor.

To return to the sexual disorders, let us take the example of a man with erectile dysfunction. If this man lives in a Buddhist monastic community in which sexual activity is prohibited, then the consequences of erectile dysfunction could be neutral or even positive for our celibate monk because there are no limitations on his activities and participation in the religious community. Indeed, our monk may even feel positive about the erectile dysfunction because it may reduce the sexual temptation or conflict in one who believes in celibacy (a personal facilitator for dealing with the "disorder"). In contrast, let's say that the erectile dysfunction occurs in a male film star who lives in Beverley Hills and whose screen image is virile and macho. Our unnamed star may develop considerable relationship problems, feelings of shame, and depression, with considerable limitations on activities and participation. Perhaps our star's problem may be relieved by the use of Viagra, or perhaps no such easy physical solution is available to solve what may be a problem that is psychological in origin. The point about a sexual "disorder" such as erectile dysfunction is that it all depends on the range of factors that have been highlighted in the ICF as to whether or not there are any consequent impairments or restrictions on functioning. Our overall proposal in this book, therefore, is that although we suggest that the ICD and DSM atheoretical classification systems be replaced with our DEC system, the framework for a biopsychosocial approach that is taken by the ICF model nevertheless provides a rich understanding of the context in which these disorders occur.

The outline of the sexual disorders in Table 4.3 also includes a category of overactivity of sexual functioning as a possible source of disorder, especially in the context of societal norms and values. However, the history and societal views on hypersexuality provide yet another remarkable story. The DSM-5 (American Psychiatric Association, 2013) no longer includes a category of hypersexuality, though ICD-10 (World Health

Organization, 1992) has the category of "Excessive sexual drive" (F52.7). The research criteria for excessive sexual drive in ICD-10 state the following:

> No research criteria are attempted for this category. Researchers studying this category are recommended to design their own criteria (World Health Organization, 1992, p. 120).

The problem of criteria for hypersexuality stated in ICD-10 perhaps sums up something of the difficulties with this diagnosis that have led DSM to sidestep it. Let us consider the example of the diagnosis of nymphomania. Although historians are unclear about the first use of the actual term nymphomania, a significant milestone was the publication in 1771 (translated into English in 1775) by an obscure French doctor, M. D. T. de Bienville, who appropriately seems to have been living in Amsterdam at the time, of the book *Nymphomania, or a Dissertation Concerning the Furor Uterinus*. As we noted in Chapter 1 on the history of psychiatry, from at least the time of Plato the problem of the "wandering uterus," or hysteria, with its origins in unrequited sexuality, had been widely discussed and had also given rise to the term *furor uterinus*, i.e., the uterine fury used in de Bienville's title. The idea of nymphomania seems to have fitted with the Enlightenment view that women were less rational than men and more vulnerable to their passions, so the term used by de Bienville has been popular ever since, certainly by comparison with its male equivalent, *satyriasis*, which few people would recognize (see Groneman, 2000). Nymphomania was therefore included as a diagnosis in DSM-1, but by DSM-III-R it had been dropped, at least in part because of the work of some famous twentieth-century sexologists. For example, the work of Alfred Kinsey on sexuality in men and women demonstrated the considerable range, variety, and frequency found within "normal" sexual activity; it was suggested that a definition for hypersexuality could be "someone who has more sex than you do." The founder of rational emotive behavior therapy, Albert Ellis, commented in a book on clinical work with so-called nymphomaniacs that none of his clients had ever met the diagnostic definition but were simply women who enjoyed their sexuality and the diagnosis was therefore irrelevant (Ellis and Sagarin, 1965). It therefore seems clear that taking a normative approach to sexual activity, such as a statistical definition of three standard deviations above or below the population mean, could be used as an approach by desperate diagnosticians to make diagnoses of hypo- and hypersexuality. DSM has at least avoided the trap of hypersexuality, even if it is still bothered by hyposexuality.

The paraphilic disorders, that is, disorders of inappropriate sexuality, as summarized in Table 4.3, are for some unknown reason given a separate chapter in DSM from the sexual disorders. The list ranges from fetishisms, to transvestism, to the pedophilias, which thereby raises the crucial (but difficult to resolve) issue of the overlap between criminality and legal definitions of "disorder," and the medical and biopsychosocial approaches to diagnosis. These issues were raised in Chapter 2 when we considered the definition of "legal insanity," which might or might not be related to diagnosis. Let us take as a first example the DSM-5 (American Psychiatric Association, 2013) paraphilia of transvestic disorder which has the following two key diagnostic criteria:

> A: Over a period of at least 6 months, recurrent and intense sexual arousal from cross-dressing, as manifested by fantasies, urges, or behaviors.

> B: The fantasies, sexual urges, or behaviors cause clinically significant distress or impairment in social, occupational, or other important areas of functioning (American Psychiatric Association, 2013, p. 702).

The problem for this disorder is in what counts as "cross-dressing" (e.g., a man wearing women's clothes), because gender-defined clothing is largely arbitrary and varies considerably with culture and historical period. Thus, in any historical period men can be found wearing the equivalent of dresses and other "female" garments, and women can be found wearing the equivalent of trousers or other "male" garments. When you live in a culture in which men wear skirts (kilts) as a statement of male national pride, the definition of "cross-dressing" begins to blur, highlighting the arbitrariness of such diagnoses. Indeed, the example of homosexuality that we considered in detail in Chapter 2 provides the prime example of how the legal, the religious, and the diagnostic need to be carefully separated. In the UK homosexuality was classified as a criminal activity until 1967, when it was decriminalized, even though it continued as a diagnostic category in DSM until 1980. Moreover, some religions still see homosexuality as contrary to the "will of god(s)" and it is therefore proscribed and seen as sinful. When all three systems, the legal, the religious, and the medical, attacked homosexuality as a criminal and sinful act with a medical diagnosis it is surely no surprise that many homosexual individuals were extremely distressed to the point of meeting Criterion B above with impairment in social and other functioning. With the paraphilias, therefore, it is the consequences of social values, as instantiated in legal and religious codes of practice, that are the primary source of distress for the individual. Similar to the wide variations in the frequency of sexuality, the variations in the objects of sexuality must also be broadened and tolerated, that is, when these activities do not involve imposition on a non-consenting or other vulnerable individual.

A more difficult example than the paraphilias is that of pedophilia. Again we have to raise the issue of cultural and historical variations to which diagnoses have to be sensitive. For example, in some cultures the allowed age of marriage can be unrestricted following traditional tribal and religious patterns. In the Sudan the age of marriage is defined as puberty, so long as both parties are willing (retrieved from <http://www.law.emory.edu/ifl/legal/sudan.htm> on July 10, 2013). The Yemen allows marriage at any age, but officially sex within child marriage is not permitted until puberty. Even the Vatican under Catholic Canon Law allows girls to be married from the age of 14 upwards (retrieved from <http://www.vatican.va> on July 10, 2013). One of the problems for the definition of pedophilia, therefore, is that it necessitates a *legal* definition rather than a *medical* definition. The argument is not that there is a problem with legal categories such as pedophilia, because society needs such rules (for example defining different speed limits for different types of roads, the exceeding of which is a criminal offence). The fact is that some of the paraphilias are incorrectly considered as medical diagnostic categories in classification systems such as DSM and ICD, when they are actually legally defined categories rather than medical ones. As a minimum, therefore, the classification systems should acknowledge that these categories are not medical diagnoses. A further comparison would be the way that Catholic Canon Law forbids sex between a priest and a woman even though that is a perfectly legal action in most secular jurisdictions. Thus a priest engaging in sex is not a sign of a medical dysfunction, even though it is prohibited under Canon Law and has serious consequences for the perpetrator. In summary, therefore, Table 4.3 in its overview of the sexual disorders includes the category of "inappropriate sexual behavior" but with the cautionary note that the definitions of "inappropriate" are more often legal rather than medical.

Sleep Disorders

Table 4.4 presents a summary categorization of the sleep disorders, again divided into "under" and "over" following the patterns already provided for the eating, elimination, and sexual disorders. There are a wide range of factors that can contribute to the different types of sleep disturbance, including a range of medical conditions that can lead to various forms of under- or oversleeping in which we would include disruption

Table 4.4: Drive–emotion–cognition analysis of sleep disorders.

Drive		Emotion	Cognition
Sleep	Under	Anxiety Excitement	Control Expectancy
	Over	Depression	Withdrawal

to the normal sleep pattern. Thus, breathing-related sleep disorders such as sleep apnea will be excluded from the current list of psychological disorders even though they are included in DSM because they are primarily the result of factors such as the distribution of fat around the neck in obese middle-aged men. Of course, the sleep disorders have general consequences for functioning and quality of life throughout the day as well as the night, but the focus here will be on those sleep disorders that are not simply the consequence of a medical condition. We will also discuss conditions that can occur during sleep, such as nightmares, and sleep behavior disorders, such as sleepwalking, especially because these can be associated with other psychological disorders.

The insomnias cover a variety of disruptions to the normal sleep pattern, including difficulty with sleep onset, difficulty maintaining sleep with frequent awakenings, and early morning awakening in which the person is unable to get back to sleep. While anybody can experience disruption to sleep once in a while, such as because of excitement before Christmas or other special events, it is the repeated and regular occurrence of insomnia that takes it into the category of a disorder, particularly because of its impact on daytime social and occupational functioning which can be severely disturbed because of constant feelings of sleepiness and poor concentration. Again, there is always an element of arbitrariness to the definitions; for example, DSM-5 defines sleep-onset insomnia as occurring when there is difficulty initiating sleep for at least 20–30 minutes, with similar figures being used for failure to maintain sleep and early morning wakening (awakening occurring before the normal wakening time).

There are a variety of emotion and cognitive factors that can contribute to the insomnias, not least that eventually worry about insomnia itself can form a vicious cycle that makes the problem of sleep even more difficult (e.g., Morin and Espie, 2003). That is, other worries such as about problems with work or relationships may initially cause the person to stay awake, but in turn these problems may be supplanted or be joined by the worry about not sleeping itself. Equally, waking during the night or early morning can be accompanied by a bout of worry about these other types of problems, but then the awakening itself can become the source of the worry that contributes to the maintenance of the problem. Interventions to overcome insomnia, such as those devised by Colin Espie and his colleagues (e.g., Morin and Espie, 2003), target aspects of "sleep hygiene" that include how to deal with worry and rumination. An additional problem is that the continued disruption to nighttime sleep and the feelings of daytime sleepiness often mean that people start napping during the day, which can further contribute to their inability to sleep at night. Interventions for insomnia therefore include an assessment of such daytime activity with encourage-ment to sleep only at night.

The hypersomnias occur when people report sleeping for normal or longer than normal times during the night but still feel tired and lapse into periods of sleep during the day. There seem to be a range of causes of hypersomnia, including viral infec-tions, drug and alcohol use, head trauma, and disorders such as depression. A crucial distinction is made between normal "long sleepers" and hypersomnia in that long sleepers feel refreshed after sleep whereas in hypersomnia people do not experience this restorative aspect (American Psychiatric Association, 2013). An extreme and sometimes life-threatening version of the hypersomnias is the disorder of narcolepsy in which sufferers can suddenly lapse into sleep, with recurrent episodes occurring throughout the day. The condition is often accompanied by sudden loss of muscle tone, leading to unsteady gait, facial grimacing, or falling over if standing. It is not uncommon for narcolepsy sufferers to fall asleep while being medically examined, which provides a strong clue to diagnosis for the examining physician.

Sleep is also the time when dreaming occurs, though despite a long history of the study of dreams, their actual function is still unclear. Freud (1900) famously proposed that dreams were the "royal road to the unconscious" in that dreams are typically a form of wish-fulfillment that incorporate residues of the previous day. However, Freud observed that one must be careful to distinguish between the *manifest* content of the dream, which can often seem bizarre and puzzling, and the *latent* content, which, although its meaning may be disguised from the dreamer, may become meaningful with careful analysis and reflection. So, you may well have dreamt that you were rising up fast through the air in a hot air balloon, when suddenly the balloon burst and you fell rapidly back down to earth. As any psychoanalyst will tell you, what the dream really means is that you clearly have considerable anxieties about your sexual perfor-mance. Just as with the rest of Freud's work, there have been considerable criticisms of his dream theory, even though some dreams can be of a Freudian nature. More recent dream theories have included Francis Crick's random neural activity theory (see Crick, 1994), in which dreams are simply a by-product of the random firing of neurons during sleep. Such a biologically reductionist theory is not appealing to a psychologist because it denies any possible function of the process of dreaming. A more interesting theory has been presented by Bill Domhoff (e.g., Domhoff, 2003); he argues that dreams are not significantly different from waking thought, but reflect the activity of a top-down schematic or "conceptual" system which is active both dur-ing wakefulness and during sleep. Indeed, during wakefulness we often daydream and mind-wander in a manner that is akin to dreaming during sleep. According to

Domhoff, therefore, the concerns and goals that drive our waking thought and activity are exactly those that provide the conceptual content of our dreams.

Sometimes our dreams can become disturbing and cause disruptions to sleep, though at the same time it is not absolutely correct to list them in the category of sleep disorders. Following the Domhoff (2003) analysis of dreams as the functioning of a top-down cognitive system working with the reduced levels of perceptual input that occur during sleep, we will return to the overlap between dreams, delusions, and hallucinations in Chapter 7 when we examine a number of linked disorders for which dreams provide a window into the blurring between the functional and the dysfunctional. That said, we should nevertheless note that nightmares are most likely to occur during rapid eye movement (REM) sleep and typically lead to awakening because of danger to self or significant others that occurs with intense feelings of anxiety and other intense emotions. The prevalence of nightmares seems to increase through childhood into adolescence, particularly around puberty at the ages of 10 to 13 (American Psychiatric Association, 2013). Nightmares can be a feature of post-traumatic stress, so the higher incidence of nightmares in adult women may be linked to higher rates of trauma.

A second category of disorder that can occur during sleep is that of sleep behavior disorders in which the individual may carry out complex actions, sometimes referred to under the generic term "sleepwalking," accompanied by vocalization. Occasionally, the problem can lead to injury to the individual or a bed partner. A client of mine reported that he was staying in a room on the fourth floor in a hotel in Switzerland and began dreaming that he was trapped in a cave that was blocked by a large rock which had fallen into the exit passageway. In fact, two days before he had seen the film *Sanctum* directed by Alister Grierson and released in 2011 in which such a scene actually occurs. However, when my client finally awoke he found himself about to climb through a window in his hotel room, a fall from which would have undoubtedly killed him. When he woke he also found that while still asleep he had carefully moved a table from in front of the window without spilling a glass of water or knocking over the lamp, both of which were still standing securely on the table in its new position. More generally, such complex behaviors can include eating while asleep, attempted sexual behavior, and night terrors with possible violent behavior. The *Guardian* newspaper (November 20, 2009) reported the case of a father of two and devoted husband, Brian Thomas, who strangled his wife Christine while they were both asleep on holiday in their camper van in west Wales. Brian had been dreaming that a boy racer had broken into their van and was fighting with him, but when he awoke he found that he had killed his wife of 40 years. The jury at Swansea Crown Court eventually found him not guilty because he had suffered

The SPAARS model of emotion

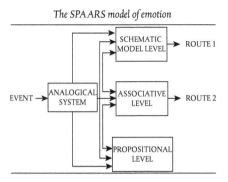

Fig. 4.2. The SPAARS model for one type of somatic symptom problem. Reproduced from Mick Power, Cognitive psychopathology: The role of emotion, *Análise Psicológica*, 27(2), Figure 4 © 2009 Instituto Superior de Psicologia Aplicada, with permission.

from "night terrors" for most of his life and on this especially tragic occasion had acted in a state of "automatism."

Somatic Symptom Disorders

Somatic symptoms are of course part of the presentation of most psychological disorders; thus, when experiencing depression, someone may have appetite disturbance and abdominal pain, or when feeling anxious they might have heart palpitations and headaches. However, there is a special category of somatic problems, illustrated by means of the SPAARS model in Figure 4.2, in which there is chronic activation of the analogical-associative system but the relevant schematic models are along the lines of rejection, inhibition, or denial of the presence or impact of the low-level chronic activation (we will consider other possibilities later). The source of this activation is likely to be an unresolved or irresolvable situation in which the person is involved, but the most predominant style of emotion regulation is, within the Phillips and

Table 4.5: Drive–emotion–cognition analysis of somatic symptoms.

Drive	Emotion	Cognition
Survival drives	Anxiety	Denial/rejection Somatization
Social drives	Shame Anxiety etc.	Denial/rejection Somatization

Power (2007) approach, that of so-called internal dysfunctional emotion regulation strategies, which are likely to have been learned at an early age.

Table 4.5 develops the SPAARS analysis further to consider somatic symptom disorders within the DEC framework. These disorders could arise from a variety of activated drives, but it is likely that those to do with social and physical survival, including the attachment drive, are a primary source of such activation and are likely to begin early in life and provide at minimum an underlying vulnerability and emotion regulation style in the face of later chronic stressors in life. The continual threat to attachment and survival drives is likely to generate chronic levels of anxiety and other emotions at an automatic low level within the system, which, if not dealt with appropriately, can have an impact on a variety of physiological systems such as the gastrointestinal and immune systems. We will return to a more detailed consideration of the attachment system and its disorders in Chapter 5 when we consider the social drives, so the focus in this section will primarily be on the range of somatic symptoms themselves and how they might best be conceptualized.

The main group of somatic symptom disorders include a range of possible somatic symptoms and a range of distressing emotions and beliefs about those symptoms, as shown in the DEC analysis in Table 4.5. As DSM-5 (American Psychiatric Association, 2013) now emphasizes in comparison with earlier DSMs, it is not simply the symptoms themselves but the accompanying thoughts and emotions about those symptoms that characterize the somatic symptom diagnosis. These symptoms can sometimes be relatively normal or common physical sensations, but they come to signify something more serious for the individual; for example the person whose mother died from bowel cancer who subsequently becomes hypersensitive to bowel sensations. In chronic pain, a combination of somatic, emotion, and cognitive factors may lead the person to alter their lifestyle dramatically but in the process increase the perpetuation of the pain. From a clinical perspective, vulnerability factors such as depression, anxiety, and insecure attachment may counteract any resources of resilience to predispose to increased pain and distress. Both resilience and vulnerability factors are likely to operate via coping and emotion regulation strategies, the effectiveness of which is largely context dependent. In some circumstances however, synchrony between pain and affect might be actually beneficial, and a lack of coherence might result in increased suffering (Dima et al., 2013).

The classification systems tend to distinguish between the somatic symptom disorders and hypochondriasis (also known as illness anxiety or health anxiety), but the same emotion-cognition processes appear to be common to both. That is, the differentiation between hypochondriasis and somatic symptom disorder may simply depend on the clinician's judgment about the extent to which the somatic symptom is actually present, with judgments that the symptom is absent or only mild leading to a diagnosis of illness anxiety or hypochondriasis, respectively. The overlap between the two sensibly implies that a broader category of somatic symptom disorder is more useful than narrower categories. In these cases there may be extensive medical procedures that fail to detect any illness, but the individual persists in the belief that there is a yet-to-be-detected illness and does not feel reassured by the procedures that have been negative. Continuous self-examination of the suspected source of the illness occurs, with repeated checking the body for signs of illness. The long chronic course of such disorders can often lead to considerable strain within families and avoidance of the affected individual.

The classification systems also highlight the category of the conversion disorders, in which neurological sensory or motor systems are affected in a manner that is not consistent with the organization of such systems anatomically. For example, an area of weakness or paralysis that is not compatible with the neuromuscular structure for a particular limb or other part of the body. The conversion disorders have a notable history, beginning with the concept of hysteria developed by the ancient Greeks, as discussed in Chapter 1. Indeed some of the early Christian miracles reported in the Bible and elsewhere are likely to have been cures of conversion disorders (Power, 2012). In more recent times, interest in hysteria and the conversion disorders rapidly increased in the nineteenth century with the work of Charcot and Janet and Freud. Under the influence of Charcot, Freud initially experimented with hypnosis as a treatment for hysteria, but then abandoned this approach for the psychoanalytic "free association" technique when one of his patients, Elizabeth von R, requested that he stopped interrupting her in order to hypnotize her when she got to the most interesting and emotional parts of her therapy (Gay, 1988). Freud was originally trained as a neurologist, and it was the anatomically puzzling conversion symptoms that he came across in his neurological practice that led him first to use hypnosis and then psychoanalysis to both understand and treat such symptoms. The influence of this history can be seen in the retention of the category "conversion disorder" as a separate diagnosis in DSM-5 (American Psychiatric Association, 2013), even though it seems unnecessary to distinguish these functional neurological symptoms from the range of other somatic symptoms which inevitably involve sensory and motor neuronal systems. Experiences of dissociation and depersonalization are also common in the conversion disorders, but these phenomena will be dealt with in more detail in Chapter 7. A number of specifically named conversion disorders have accumulated over the years such as dysphonia (reduced speech volume), dysarthria (problems with speech articulation), globus (lump in the throat), diplopia (double vision), and psychogenic seizures, discussed in the next paragraph.

Psychogenic or "non-epileptic" attacks provide an interesting example of the conversion disorders. DSM-5 notes that such attacks peak in people in their 20s and are more common in women. Although it is difficult to distinguish non-epileptic from epileptic attacks, because the person is unlikely to be connected to an EEG machine during the attack, certain discriminating features are present that include resistance to opening the eyes if they are closed, biting only of the tip of the tongue, and the absence of complex motor automatisms, all of which can be indicators of the non-epileptic nature of the seizure. The psychological origin of such seizures means that they are associated with higher rates of childhood abuse and neglect, with recent significant life events, and with patterns of emotion regulation that are associated with increased dissociation and depersonalization (Reuber and Elger, 2003).

A final category that the classification systems also list under the somatic disorders is that of the factitious disorders, which involve the knowingly deceptive presentation of illness in oneself (sometimes referred to as Munchausen syndrome, after the infamous baron who was a teller of tall tales, as we noted in Chapter 2) or occasionally in others such as a child (Munchausen by proxy). The diagnosis hinges on the falsification of signs and symptoms through deliberate induction or injury. However, because the sign or symptom is secondary to its induction, in contrast to DSM we propose that the factitious disorders are *not* somatic disorders but should be considered a type of social-cognitive disorder; we will therefore consider them in more detail in the next chapter (Chapter 5) when we deal with disorders of social drives. These disorders are motivated by a need for professional care and attention, or leniency from authority, and may originate in earlier positive experiences of healthcare for a genuine illness or disorder, hence the interpretation that they need to be understood as social phenomena in terms of their interpersonal function.

Although in this section we have focused on the importance of repression/denial and other internal dysfunctional emotion regulation strategies in relation to the somatic disorders (as summarized in Figure 4.2), this analysis does not assume that this is the only possible profile that can lead to such disorders. For example, in chronic overwhelmingly stressful situations, in particular those in which people feel trapped and humiliated, there may be a whole variety of different somatic symptoms that come to be part of the body's response to chronic stress. A common disorder such as depression includes a range of potential somatic symptoms in addition to the cognitive, emotional, and interpersonal ones (Cheung and Power, 2012), but the difference from the specifically somatic disorders that have been considered in this section is that disorders such as depression include dysphoric mood, anhedonia, etc., that are not part of the presentation in the somatic disorders in which the cognitive–emotional focus is on the meaning and implication of the somatic symptoms themselves. Thus, in depression experiences of pain, abdominal problems, and so on, are typically seen by the sufferer as accompaniments to their depression, whereas in the somatic disorders these symptoms are the focus of the disorder with their interpretation as signs of major illness.

Summary and Conclusions

In this chapter we started with the exciting possibility that modern genetics may eventually reveal important gene–environment interactions in which under some environmental conditions certain genes may give rise to advantage but under other conditions may be disadvantageous. Such an approach may eventually help us to understand why many psychological disorders have not disappeared but are maintained or may even be on the increase. Important differences in a child's early environment center on physical and social resources; first the young child needs sufficient nutrients and energy for physical development, but also sufficient social resources to ensure their safety and survival within the framework of secure attachment relationships. This work on gene–environment interactions is at an extremely early stage, as evidenced by the lack of relevant evidence of such interactions in relation to the disorders that can develop around the biological drives of eating, sleeping, sexuality, and more general somatic symptoms. In the context of a summary of such disorders, a warning was issued about how the imposition of social norms and values can lead to a false medical diagnosis; a classic example of this is homosexuality, which until recently was both criminalized and medicalized but which has now been freed from the imposition of such inappropriate norms and values. However, at the same time norms and values can be important in terms of the definition of *legal* as opposed to medical categories, which serve the purpose of protecting individuals, especially those who are vulnerable, from being victims, in particular of sex crimes. The paraphilias thereby provide a set of legally defined categories, but these should not be confused with medical diagnostic categories.

Finally, we should note that the general DEC framework is extremely useful in helping us to understand even the most biological of the disorders that this chapter has focused on. Even if a drive disorder has arisen due to a primarily biologically related reason, the person's own emotion and cognition reactions, as well as those of significant others and society around them, have important consequences for the maintenance and course of such disorders. For example, in the somatic disorders a specific but genuine somatic symptom may come to signify a lethal disease in the mind of the sufferer, whose consequent lifestyle changes may in fact increase the likelihood of the feared disease occurring rather than decrease it. The management of all of the disorders summarized in this chapter is therefore just as likely to include the management of emotion and cognition as it is to include the management of their somatic underpinnings.

5

DISORDERS OF SOCIAL DRIVES

Sanity calms, but madness is more interesting

John Russell

Introduction

We will simplify the world of social functioning with the proposal that there are a set of social drives, akin to the biological drives considered in Chapter 4, which provide the starting point for socio-emotional development in the child, but which can then take a number of different courses depending on a variety of influences through life. We will consider work on initial temperamental differences in childhood and how these can interact with different parenting and attachment styles—providing a further example of the gene–environment interactions that we flagged up in Chapter 4. The important point from this work is that even with the same starting point the outcomes can be functional or dysfunctional according to different environmental influences. Next we will examine the burgeoning area of attachment and attachment styles and how dysfunctional attachment styles may be precursors for a wide variety of disorders. We will also consider work on a variety of personality-type disorders that are apparent in childhood, including conduct disorders and psychopathy (the "callous unemotional type"), which cut across disorders of cognition and emotion but which include important dysfunctional social relating.

We will then consider some of the neurodevelopmental disorders, for example autistic spectrum disorder (ASD), which again cut across the cognition and emotion disorders but which involve very clear impairments in social functioning. These neurodevelopmental disorders can lead to excessive delays in the development of appropriate social functioning, and in some individuals adequate social functioning may never be achieved. In contrast, there are a variety of acquired disorders, for example head trauma or the dementia-related pathologies later in life, in which previously adequate socio-emotional functioning subsequently deteriorates and may be lost. These acquired disorders will be discussed in detail in Chapter 7, but it is important to note that they also have considerable consequences for socio-emotional functioning.

Temperament

The modern impetus for the study of child temperament came from publications by Thomas, Chess and colleagues in the 1960s about their longitudinal study of child development in New York (e.g., Thomas et al., 1963). This early research pointed to how initial differences in children's abilities to regulate their emotions and their responsiveness to stimulation had a significant impact on subsequent social development. Although Thomas and Chess identified nine possible dimensions on which children differ, subsequent work on the empirical and conceptual overlap of these dimensions has led to the identification of three major temperament dimensions (Sanson et al., 2004):

1. Reactivity or negative emotionality—a high level of emotionality especially in response to new or to distressing situations with reactions such as anger, irritability, fearfulness, and low mood.
2. Self-regulation—this capacity includes the ability to control attention in addition to the control and regulation of emotional reactions.
3. Inhibition or sociability—a dimension that refers to a tendency to withdraw versus to be open to sociability.

Jerome Kagan and his colleagues (e.g., Kagan, 1998) have suggested that part of the biological basis for such differences in temperament may relate to the sensitivity or threshold level of reactivity of the amygdala to arousal, with heritability of the traits being at around about 0.5. The main measures of temperament are based on parent-completed questionnaires or direct observation of children.

Much of the research on temperament has been designed around a main effects-type model such that the early presence of a particular temperament trait is associated with a later behavioral outcome. For example, Kagan and colleagues (Kagan, 1998) followed a sample of more than 400 4-month-old babies until they were over 7 years of age and found that those children rated as "inhibited" as babies were more likely to show internalizing problems such as anxiety symptoms at age 7 (45%) than those who were uninhibited as babies (15%). Similarly, externalizing problems such as later aggressive behavior, conduct disorder, and substance abuse were more likely for those babies who were higher on negative emotionality in comparison with those low on this trait.

Instead of looking for major effects of temperament across time, one of the more interesting lines of recent work has been to look for interactions between temperament and key social–environmental factors such as parenting style, along the lines of the gene–environment interactions that we have referred to throughout this book. In a study of 5–6-year-old children Paterson and Sanson (1999) studied interactions between temperament and parenting and found that "poor fit," such as the parents reporting on a child's behavior that they found unacceptable and bothersome, predicted the presence of externalizing behavior problems in the children, with poor parenting being reflected by factors such as low warmth and high punishment. A small but fascinating study by DeVries (1984) reported on temperament in a group of Masai children, a pastoral people who live in central Kenya and Tanzania in Africa. DeVries originally found the same range of "easy" and "difficult" temperament styles reported by Thomas and Chess in US children. However, when a small sample of these children were later followed up after there had been an extreme drought and famine, it was unexpectedly found that more of the children with a difficult temperament had survived than children with an easy temperament. DeVries speculated that a combination of factors may have led to the beneficial effects of a difficult childhood temperament during famine and drought, including a parenting style that encouraged warrior-like aggressiveness in the children and the likelihood that the more difficult children were given more of the limited food supplies because of their demanding nature.

One of the more recent lines of work on child temperament has revolved around attempts to integrate studies of childhood temperament and adult personality, because it is likely that the temperaments of children should provide the later grounds for the differences in adult personality. For a number of years, the dominant model of adult personality has been the five-factor model (FFM) of Costa and McCrae (e.g., McCrae and Costa, 1987), which includes the key personality dimensions of neuroticism, extraversion, conscientiousness, agreeableness, and openness to experience. There have now been several attempts to map the different temperament systems conceptually onto the FFM (e.g., Caspi and Shiner, 2006; De Pauw and Mervielde, 2010), and although these integrations have arrived at somewhat different proposals there is nevertheless sufficient overlap to warrant further empirical and conceptual work. However, we recall the problems discussed in Chapter 2 that the designers of DSM-5 struggled with in their attempts to combine the dimensional approach of the FFM of normal personality with the traditional DSM diagnostic approach of categories of personality disorders. In the end, the designers of DSM-5 were unable to agree and so handed the problem over to the future designers of DSM-6 and the current group working on ICD-11. The point is that the future integrations should attempt to cover not just childhood temperament and adult personality, but also personality disorder. We will consider some of the conundrums of personality and personality disorder later in this chapter.

In summary, to begin our review of possible disorders of social drives we have begun with the issue of possible different starting temperaments that may interact with different social environments to the extent that apparently dysfunctional traits may actually be advantageous in certain environments, as in the study of mortality in Masai children. These important gene–environment interactions, although very poorly understood, may provide some understanding of why the range of psychological problems in children and adults does not diminish across evolutionary time— in fact some disorders appear to be increasing. The key point is that in certain social environments these so-called disadvantageous traits may instead be advantageous. We briefly considered aspects of parenting and how these might interact with temperament traits, but we now turn to the area of attachment research which can offer a more detailed understanding of such gene–environment interactions.

Attachment

Perhaps one of the fastest-growing fields of research in recent years has been in the area of attachment. Work on attachment began mainly with John Bowlby after the Second World War, and we will focus on that here—but as noted in Chapter 3 the work of Harry Harlow with young rhesus monkeys in the 1950s also had an important influence. Harlow demonstrated that simple behavioral reinforcement models of mother–child relationships were inadequate to explain the baby monkey's preference for a "terrycloth mother" that was tactilely more similar to the real mother than a mother made from wire who actually provided milk (e.g., Harlow, 1959).

John Bowlby's work began with a report published in 1951 on behalf of the World Health Organization, *Maternal Care and Mental Health*. Following the Second World War there was considerable concern about the number of orphans in Europe and Bowlby's report had considerable influence on the way in which institutional care was provided by such institutions. In 1952 a moving documentary film made by James Robertson, *A Two-Year Old Goes to the Hospital*, powerfully summarized the painful effects that even brief separations can have on young children. At that time, however, many of Bowlby's psychoanalytic colleagues strongly opposed his ideas about the importance of the need for a primary caregiver such as the mother for each child—he is reported to have been treated as an outcast at his place of work, the Tavistock Clinic in north London, then under the control of Melanie Klein and her followers.

Bowlby subsequently developed attachment theory by drawing together his own work on maternal deprivation with the newly developing areas of ethology, developmental psychology, and cognitive science, to show how an innately based attachment system develops within the primary attachment relationship, typically to the mother, in the early childhood years. Bowlby's landmark trilogy was *Attachment and Loss* the first volume of which was published in 1969. Bowlby proposed that the young child develops internal working models of key relationships that then have a strong influence on psychosocial development and on relationships both in childhood and through into adult life.

One of the important developments made by Bowlby's PhD student, Mary Ainsworth, was the so-called strange situation test in which a child was briefly separated from his or her caregiver and then subsequently reunited. The range of behaviors and reactions observed in the child could then be coded into secure versus insecure attachment types, with the insecure attachment style being further divided into anxious attachment or avoidant attachment. Mary Main subsequently added a fourth type, that of disorganized attachment, which has been widely accepted by attachment theorists.

Table 5.1 presents a simplified account of the possible interactions between temperament and attachment, while noting that so far there has only been limited relevant research because attachment and temperament represent two distinct research traditions. The temperament dimensions have been simplified into two categories of "easy" and "difficult," in line with a number of temperament researchers who have used such a simplification in their analyses of outcomes. Similarly, for the sake of presentation the attachment dimensions have been simplified into "secure" versus "insecure." The important point is that outcome depends on the interaction of the two factors rather than on the main effects of any one factor; for example, the "difficult" temperament might actually lead to enhanced outcome in the context of a secure attachment, mirroring the effects noted for the Masai children discussed earlier. However, it is possible that insecure attachment could have a worse outcome when it interacts with difficult temperament, but in the context of an easy temperament there

Table 5.1: The interaction of temperament and attachment.

	Attachment style	
	Secure	Insecure
Easy temperament	Good outcome	Recovery?
Difficult temperament	Good outcome?	Poor outcome

may be increased possibility of recovery, especially with later good relationships that can make up for an initial insecure attachment (see, e.g., Rutter 1981).

As we noted above, the two traditionally separate research traditions, child temperament and attachment, have only recently begun to converge in order to study possible interactions between the two. Porter (2009) reported a study of children aged 35 to 58 months who were assessed on temperament (measures of shyness, impulsivity, and social withdrawal) and attachment and peer network size in order to investigate how these factors predicted different types of play, such as solitary versus social play, which are predictive of later social development and risk of psychopathology. It was found that a multidimensional approach taking account of both temperament and attachment factors provided the best prediction of type of play. Booth-LaForce and Oxford (2008) reported on the large US National Institute of Child Health and Human Development (NICHD) longitudinal study, which included a sample of 1092 children whose social interactions in school were followed from the first to the sixth grades. From within this larger sample, the authors identified two key social development pathways, one in which the children showed *increasing* social withdrawal across the time of the study and the other in which initially withdrawn children showed *decreasing* social withdrawal. Structural equation modeling showed that the decreasing group were initially characterized by insensitive parenting, less secure attachment, and shyness temperamentally, but that the school peer relationships gradually began to improve social functioning and to reduce social withdrawal across time. Similarly, the *increasing* social withdrawal group were also found to be characterized by insensitive parenting and less secure attachment, but temperamentally they were more dysregulated, especially with poor inhibitory control, which led to immature and socially incompetent behavior.

A recent study of distress in infants undergoing venipuncture was reported by Wolff et al. (2011). The study involved 246 infants aged approximately 14 months who had previously been assessed with the Ainsworth strange situation test for attachment security and whose parents had rated them on a variety of infant temperament scales. The children were rated for distress during the blood sampling procedure on behaviors such as crying, resisting, seeking parental support, and inability to use distraction through play. The results showed that none of the individual temperament traits nor the insecure attachment categories predicted level of distress when analyzed separately (apart from a small effect of disorganized attachment); however, the infant group that showed both disorganized attachment and higher temperamental fear showed the highest levels of distress during the procedure.

The studies of temperament–attachment relationships that have been considered so far have considered outcomes such as social withdrawal or distress which can at best only be risk factors for the later development of psychopathology. There is of course a considerable inferential leap to go from increased distress at 14 months or social withdrawal and solitary play at 48 months to the psychological disorders of later in life. Nevertheless, one or two studies have now tried to begin to assess longitudinally what the contribution of these gene–environment interactions might be for later development and psychopathology. For example, a study reported by Brumariu and Sterns (2013) included further analyses from the US NICHD study mentioned earlier in which they investigated children's attachment patterns at 15 and 36 months, temperament at 54 months, peer competence and emotion regulation at early school age, and then anxiety symptoms in pre-adolescence in the fifth and sixth grades at school (typically 9–12 years old). Their findings showed that while both temperament and attachment security predicted later anxiety, these effects were moderated by peer competence and emotion regulation, findings that point to the impact of the interaction of temperament and attachment factors on developing socio-emotional skills.

In summary, therefore, all of these recent studies point to exciting areas of research in child development and how factors such as temperament, parenting, and attachment interact. At present we know that these factors interact to impact on the development of social functioning, as Peter Fonagy and his colleagues at University College London have emphasized in their studies of attachment and mentalization skills (e.g., Fonagy et al., 2003). Problems in socio-emotional functioning, such as in the capacity for mentalization, create risk and vulnerability for later development and may interact with subsequent adversity to lead to a wide range of different psychological disorders. The subtle combinations of parenting–attachment–temperament may well be differentially predictive of different types of adolescent and adult psychopathology, but the research at present can only point to a more general risk for almost all later psychopathology. For example, in a long-term study of psychosis, Myhrman et al. (1996) reported the findings from a prospective study of 11,017 pregnant women in a birth cohort study in northern Finland. Around the sixth or seventh months of their pregnancy the women were asked whether their pregnancies were wanted or unwanted. An analysis of Finnish hospital records 28 years later showed that whereas the rate of schizophrenia was 0.7% for the wanted pregnancies it increased to 1.5% for the unwanted pregnancies, with an odds ratio of 2.4 of unwanted to wanted remaining even after the authors controlled for a variety of possible confounding sociodemographic factors. Of course, such findings now require further longitudinal studies that can tease apart the various gene–environment interactions. For now, the best we can say is that problems with attachment and parenting are likely to interact with temperamental factors to impair the development of socio-emotional functioning, which in turn will increase the risk for the subsequent development of a variety of psychological disorders. In this context, we will now go on to consider personality disorders, which have a considerable impact on socio-emotional disorders, while noting that almost all psychological disorders are possible consequences of these early gene–environment interactions.

Personality Disorders—and the Magic Number Five

The past decades of research on normal personality have coalesced in the proposal of the so-called big five personality traits. Hans Eysenck in earlier work highlighted three higher-order factors of personality that included extraversion, neuroticism, and psychoticism (e.g., Eysenck and Eysenck, 1985). These three dimensions combined together, Eysenck argued, such that high values of extraversion, neuroticism, and psychoticism produced different types of personality disorder. However, one of the criticisms of Eysenck's "psychoticism" dimension is that it is mislabeled and is more reflective of an impulsive, unempathic, and antisocial type than having anything to do with a proneness to psychosis (e.g., Claridge and Davis, 2002). Subsequent work by Digman (e.g., Digman, 1990) and Costa and McCrae (1992) has established the FFM that builds on Eysenck's approach:

1. Neuroticism, for example anxiety, hostility, vulnerability.
2. Extraversion, for example sociability, warmth, excitement seeking, positive emotions.
3. Openness to experience, for example fantasy, ideas, feelings.
4. Agreeableness, for example trust, altruism, compliance.
5. Conscientiousness, for example order, dutifulness, self-discipline.

Although it might seem sensible to base a classification system for personality disorders on the well-researched area of normal personality, as we discussed in detail in Chapter 2, systems such as DSM have taken an atheoretical approach to the issue of personality disorder based on committee consensus. However, for DSM-5 there was a preliminary attempt to draw together the diagnostic categorical approach and the FFM dimensional approach, but the Personality Disorders Work Group failed to reach agreement and a number of leading personality theorists resigned in protest (Emmelkamp and Power, 2012). Nevertheless, DSM-5 presents *both* possible approaches to personality disorder: first, the traditional list of 10 personality disorders that have been imported from DSM-IV are repeated in DSM-5 with the recommendation that they continue to be used; second, an alternative five-trait dimensional approach based on the FFM model and from which a set of putative personality disorders have been derived is also presented. We will return to these two alternative approaches later in the section, but before we do we will take a short digression into the "magic number five," which seems to keep reoccurring with five basic emotions, the five senses, five personality traits, and even DSM-5. OK, so DSM-5 is obviously a coincidence, but it is worth stopping to consider whether or not the five basic emotions and five personality traits might be sheer happenstance.

The basic emotions approach was presented in detail in Chapter 3, where it was summarized that the basic emotions that have been most widely agreed upon and included in almost all modern lists are the five emotions of anger, sadness, fear, disgust, and happiness. These emotions are "basic" according to a range of criteria, though we have drawn the list from the work of Oatley and Johnson-Laird (1987). As a further aside, we might note that the number "five" for basic emotions has interesting precedents; for example, some 2500 years ago in his classic *The Art of War* Sun-Tzu noted in passing:

> There are but five notes, and yet their permutations are more than can ever be heard.
> There are but five colours, and yet their permutations are more than ever can be seen.
> There are but five flavours, and yet their permutations are more than can ever be tasted.
> (Sun-Tzu, 2002, pp. 25–26)

Indeed, the importance of five types in Chinese extends not only to the notes, colors, and flavors commented on by Sun-Tzu, but, more importantly to the five elements or phases (wood, fire, earth, metal, water—in contrast to the *four* elements identified by the Greeks), that form the basis of Chinese medicine and Chinese martial arts, and that are taken into account in the practice of feng shui, which considers the energy flows between the five elements.

It can reasonably be asked therefore whether or not the five basic emotions and the five personality traits might in some way be connected. For example, what if the individual differences in temperamental and basic emotion starting points at birth interact with parenting styles, attachment patterns, and peer relationships and eventually lead to the different patterns of personality that become evident by adolescence and early adulthood? It would be an entirely reasonable conjecture to place socio-emotional development at the core of personality development rather than these systems being considered in isolation from each other. Table 5.2 attempts a preliminary mapping of basic emotions onto personality traits, some of which map onto each other more readily than others. From Eysenck's work on neuroticism onwards there has been a recognition that this personality trait primarily reflects different levels of anxiety (e.g., Eysenck and Eysenck, 1985). However, the FFM model has also added some hostility (anger) to this mix, so we would note possible contributions from other basic emotions such as anger to the neuroticism factor.

Table 5.2: Basic emotions and personality—possible relations.

Emotion	Personality	DSM personality disorder
Anxiety	Neuroticism	Cluster C
Anger	(Dis)Agreeableness	Cluster B
Disgust	Conscientiousness	Cluster A
Sadness	Closed/openness to experience	Cluster A
Happiness	Extraversion	Cluster A

The second personality trait in Table 5.2 is that of agreeableness/disagreeableness, which again would seem to have the clearest overlap with the basic emotion of anger, in that the hostility factor would contribute especially to disagreeableness in inter-personal relations.

The third personality trait in Table 5.2, that of conscientiousness, has perhaps a less clear overlap with the basic emotions than the previous two traits. The table therefore highlights the possible role of the basic emotion of disgust, in the sense that disgust provides much of the underpinning of the *moral* emotions such as shame and guilt (e.g., Power and Dalgleish, 2008) that may underpin the wish to be conscien-tious in relation to others. However, again it seems likely that some contribution of other basic emotions such as anxiety may play a possible role in the development of conscientiousness.

The fourth and fifth personality traits in Table 5.2 are openness to experience and extraversion. The trait of extraversion has been most linked with the positive emo-tions (Costa and McCrae, 1992), but low scores on extraversion may be somewhat associated with increased sadness, especially that extreme forms of sadness such as those seen in depression may lead to complete social withdrawal. Equally, this social withdrawal may lead to the person being more closed to experience, in contrast to happiness which is typically associated with more openness to experience, as sum-marized in Barbara Fredrickson's broaden-and-build theory (e.g., Fredrickson, 2009).

In the third column in Table 5.2 we have summarized the 10 personality disorders from DSM-IV/DSM-5 in to the three clusters that are sometimes used to summarize the DSM disorders:

Cluster A: paranoid, schizoid, and schizotypal.
Cluster B: antisocial, borderline, histrionic, and narcissistic.
Cluster C: avoidant, dependent, obsessive–compulsive.

The attempt to map these three clusters onto the five personality traits, and therefore to the five basic emotions, is only partly successful, in that Cluster C seems to have a preponderance of neuroticism and anxiety and Cluster B a preponderance of disagreeableness and anger. However, the odd/eccentric disorders of Cluster A do not seem to readily map onto the personality traits, though we have suggested the possible contributions of extraversion and openness/closedness to experience. However, we should note that although some researchers use the cluster summaries as a shorthand, there is only mixed support for the cluster groupings (American Psychiatric Association, 2013).

The alternative dimensional approach to the personality disorders presented in DSM-5 is summarized in Table 5.3. The right-hand column presents the proposed names for "personality disorder traits," which are based on the FFM but with a proposed relabeling of the five factors in order to emphasize disorder as follows:

1. Negative affectivity (versus emotional stability)—a renaming of the neuroticism personality trait under the influence of the Watson and Clark (e.g., Watson and Clark, 1992) negative affectivity proposal, which presumably reflects the fact that Lee Anna Clark was on the committee.
2. Antagonism (versus agreeableness)—a range of hostile behaviors and feelings of self-importance that put the individual at odds with others.
3. Disinhibition (versus conscientiousness)—impulsive and irresponsible behavior with risky and often self-damaging actions.
4. Psychoticism (versus lucidity)—this personality disorder trait least resembles the "big five" factor of openness to experience and therefore provides the most controversial of the proposed disorder traits. However, unlike Eysenck's

Table 5.3: Basic emotions and personality—possible relations with alternative DSM model.

Emotion	Personality	DSM-5 personality disorder trait (proposed)
Anxiety	Neuroticism	Negative affectivity
Anger	(Dis)Agreeableness	Antagonism
Disgust	Conscientiousness	Disinhibition
Sadness	Closed/openness to experience	Psychoticism
Happiness	Extraversion	Detachment

proposed psychoticism scale discussed earlier (which sounds more like the disinhibition trait), this psychoticism trait covers odd and eccentric behaviors, beliefs in unusual abilities such as mind-reading, and odd experiences including dissociation, depersonalization, and derealization.

5. Detachment (versus extraversion)—withdrawal from others, restricted socio-emotional experience, avoidance of intimacy, and suspiciousness of others.

Again, it is clear from our attempt to map from basic emotion to personality trait to personality disorder trait that there is clear cross-over, with contributions from two or more basic emotions to personality traits and two or more personality traits to personality disorder traits. It would also seem to be possible to apply the "coupling" approach, in which two or more basic emotions can become automatically linked and that we have argued applies to basic emotions (Power and Dalgleish, 2008) (see Chapter 6 for a detailed account), to the disordered personality traits, as shown in Table 5.4. Particular combinations of the coupled personality traits would then provide different types of chronic vulnerability and problems in self-development and interpersonal relations; for example, negative affectivity coupled with detachment (social withdrawal) would leave the person extremely vulnerable to experiencing periods of depression, antagonism coupled with disinhibition would be likely to lead to problems in interpersonal aggression, and so on. As with emotion coupling, it seems likely that some combinations of personality traits might be more likely to occur than others, but it would be an interesting empirical test of the model to examine such possible combinations. Despite its many shortcomings, therefore, something along the lines of this five-dimensional system that draws on the work on normal personality may provide a better starting point for the structural analysis of possible personality

Table 5.4: Possible coupling of personality traits in personality disorders.

	Negative affectivity	Antagonism	Disinhibition	Psychoticism	Detachment
Negative affectivity					
Antagonism					
Disinhibition					
Psychoticism					
Detachment					

disorders. It is hoped that such work will have made considerable progress between now and the development of DSM-6, whenever that may be. Alternatively, a possible further simplification being considered by the revision group for ICD-11 is that all personality disorders could be lumped together and simply defined by a dimension of severity. We await to see what the future holds for the personality disorders.

Neurodevelopmental Disorders

There are a large number of neurodevelopmental disorders, each of which can have a varying impact on social functioning, emotional expression, and cognitive development; these disorders could therefore be subsumed under several headings in this book—indeed different aspects of these disorders will be highlighted in different chapters. The range of disorders included under this title are general and specific intellectual disabilities, language and other communication disorders, ASD, ADHD, neurodevelopmental motor disorders including vocal tics (Tourette's syndrome), genetic disorders such as fragile X and Rett syndrome, fetal alcohol syndrome, and traumatic brain injury including congenital injury. The variety of causes of this range of disorders stretch from genetic, to immune dysfunction, to nutrition, to trauma, to infection, to toxic environmental factors. Except for the identified genetic disorders, the etiology of many of the other disorders is poorly understood and a number of disorders seem to result from a variety of possible causes.

The ASD provide a fascinating insight into the complexity of the neurodevelopmental disorders, while highlighting the significant social deficits that accompany such disorders. In one of his descriptions of the lack of affective contact in the schizophrenias, Eugen Bleuler used the term "autism" to describe a person living in their own world and not in the world of others (see the impressive book by Tantam, 2013). Leo Kanner working in Chicago, though trained in Europe, and Hans Asperger, working in Vienna, used variations on Bleuler's term to describe a group of children with extreme social difficulties. The work of Leo Kanner was better known and started the modern tradition of studying autistic disorder. The work of Hans Asperger was rediscovered by Lorna Wing in the 1970s and 1980s (e.g., Wing, 1981); she used the term "Asperger's syndrome" to refer to a group of high-functioning individuals with autistic disorder who did not present with intellectual disabilities. The well-known film *Rain Man* released in 1988, in which Dustin Hoffman plays the character Raymond Babbitt, is a portrayal of a person with Asperger's syndrome with some "autistic savant" ability (memory and calculation skills). Lorna Wing trained Dustin Hoffman in how to portray someone with Asperger's; at that time I worked in the MRC Social Psychiatry Unit where we used to listen in fascination to Lorna's stories about Dustin Hoffman's brilliant acting skills, and how she was much less impressed by Tom Cruise.

In DSM-IV (1994) autistic disorder was listed as a type of pervasive developmental disorder that also included Asperger's syndrome, Rett syndrome, and childhood disintegrative disorder as separate disorders. These are often but not always accompanied by intellectual disability (or "mental retardation" as it was termed in DSM-IV), by severe impairment in social interaction and communication skills, and by the presence of stereotyped behavior, interests, and activities, and are all typically observable in the early years of life. Lorna Wing (e.g., Wing, 1991) always emphasized a *triad* of deficits that included impaired verbal and non-verbal communication and restricted or stereotyped activities and interests, just as she also emphasized a *spectrum* of disorder that ranged from low-functioning autistic disorder to high-functioning Asperger's syndrome. This concept of a spectrum has been especially influential in recent years, such that DSM-5 has now grouped the separate disorders of DSM-IV listed above into ASD. The DSM-5 diagnostic criteria include:

A1: deficits in social–emotional reciprocity
A2: deficits in non-verbal communication
A3: deficits in developing and maintaining relationships.

There are also other important criteria in DSM-5, including restricted and repetitive interests and activities, but it is important to emphasize that the primary diagnostic criteria focus on socio-emotional functioning, which in turn leads to the question of what mechanisms might lie behind such poor functioning, a question that we will briefly consider next.

Simon Baron-Cohen (e.g., Baron-Cohen, 2003) has argued that perhaps our most important clue about the autistic spectrum is that up to 10 times more men than women suffer from these disorders—though see the work of Cordelia Fine (e.g., Fine, 2010) which is highly critical of the "hardwiring" approach of Baron-Cohen and others. Baron-Cohen has argued that differences in male versus female brains mean that while women are better at general socio-emotional skills, such as what he terms *empathizing*, men are better at skills that he terms *systemizing*; thus, a classic example of the autistic spectrum is a boy or man with good systemizing and organizing skills who is low on empathizing skills, and who is therefore impaired in social relations through poor understanding of the mental states of both himself and others. One of the features that Baron-Cohen emphasizes is that the disorder is not degenerative, and at least some proportion of sufferers may develop and continue to improve social and language skills in adulthood and find niches in certain types of work. For example, Baron-Cohen (2003) provides a very moving account of a brilliant professor of mathematics in Cambridge who clearly suffers from an autistic disorder but who nevertheless has been awarded the Fields Medal in mathematics (the mathematics equivalent of the Nobel Prize).

Research by Simon Baron-Cohen, Uta Frith, Alan Leslie, and colleagues on the so-called theory of mind (TOM) has brought autism research to the forefront in psychology and psychiatry in the past two or three decades. TOM is the capacity to set aside one's own mental state and be able to attribute a mental state to another person, the content of which can be inferred from a variety of historical and contextual clues (Baron-Cohen, 2003). In neurotypical development, TOM capacity can be seen in girls as young as 3 years, though girls tend be slightly ahead of boys. Wimmer and Perner (1983) developed a test of false beliefs known as the "Sally–Anne" task in which one of two dolls moves a ball from one box to another, unbeknownst to the first doll. The child is then asked in which box the first doll, Sally, will look for her ball—will she look where the child knows the ball to have been moved to, or will Sally look in the box where she last knew the ball to be? Neurotypical children can pass the Sally–Anne test typically between 3 and 4 years of age and a more complex second-order TOM task by the ages of 6 to 8. In contrast, individuals with ASD fail on these TOM tasks, with low-functioning individuals never likely to gain the capacity whereas higher-functioning individuals are much more likely eventually to do so (Tantam, 2013).

From the point of view of social functioning, therefore, one of the key problems that can emerge in ASD is the lack of capacity to be aware of mental states in other people, be this through TOM problems, lack of empathy, or whatever. Poor social functioning is a clear consequence of this lack of capacity for socio-emotional skills. However, TOM and empathy skills occur relatively late in development and are not observed in neurotypical children until 3 of 4 years of age, whereas parents of children with ASD (and other tests) reveal problems that are already present in their younger children even before the capacity for empathy and TOM develops. It seems likely therefore that there may be more specific problems that underlie ASD and that are evident earlier in development, though some of the consequences of these earlier developmental problems must include the delay or absence of the later more sophisticated socio-emotional skills. In this sense, the work on TOM has not answered the question of what the deficits are in ASD, but has merely demonstrated that certain earlier developmental problems contribute to later developmental delays. The crucial question therefore is what difficulties can already be observed in children with ASD prior to the TOM-type problems.

An example of a perceptual processing problem that can arise early in development and that could contribute to later socio-emotional problems in ASD could be problems with integrative holistic or gestalt perceptual processes and an emphasis on fine-grained local perceptual processes. For example, if the autistic child processed fine-grained perceptual detail but failed to integrate this detail into a holistic gestalt, a task as apparently straightforward as processing a facial stimulus would be problematic; thus, a concentration on fine-grain detail could lead to too much attention to the mouth or nose in a facial stimulus and a failure to process the eyes, thereby failing to process the overall facial percept. In fact, one of the observations that parents sometimes make about babies who go on to develop ASD is that they do not seem to give as much direct eye gaze as do neurotypical children. Such observations have led Tony Charman and colleagues (Elsabbagh et al., 2012) to show that, even as young as 6 to 10 months, children who go on later to develop autism (subsequently diagnosed at 36 months) showed different patterns of processing of faces, some of which had gaze toward the child and some of which had gaze away from the child, when compared with neurotypical children. An underlying deficit in local versus gestalt perceptual processing provides just one example of how a basic cognitive deficit could contribute to later problems in socio-emotional processing (cf. Hermelin and O'Connor, 1970).

In this section on neurodevelopmental disorders we have deliberately concentrated on the autistic spectrum because of the exciting research that has been done in this area in recent years. However, the comparative lack of work on some of the other neurodevelopmental disorders should not distract from the fact that similar aspects about developmental problems can apply across the wide range of these disorders and are likely to emerge as these disorders become the focus of research. Nevertheless, it is clear from what is known about these disorders that even when they do not impact on specific cognitive abilities, they can impact on high-level socio-emotional processes that reflect the highest levels of functioning as a consequence of our evolutionary development. Although the underlying problems may be, for example, specific issues in perceptual processing, these basic factors interact to produce the high-level consequences for social functioning that can be observed in the neurodevelopmental disorders.

Factitious Disorders

The factitious disorders are listed in DSM-5 as a type of somatic symptom disorder, which is puzzling because in fact they represent the ultimate *social* disorder in that one person deliberately attempts to deceive one or more other people into believing that he/she has a physical or psychological problem. The feigning of symptoms can be simply through self-report or it can include the deliberate induction of signs or symptoms through taking medically active substances, or through other forms of self-injury. Factitious disorder by proxy (renamed as factitious disorder imposed on another in DSM-5) involves the induction of physical and/or psychological symptoms in another individual, typically a child by a parent. As we noted earlier (see Chapters 2 and 4), the factitious disorders are sometimes referred to in Europe as Munchausen syndrome and Munchausen syndrome by proxy, after the infamous Baron von Münchhausen who was a great teller of tall stories.

Savino and Fordtran (2006) presented a series of such cases that they worked with in Baylor University Medical Centre. The first case, that of a young woman suffering from diarrhea, was initially investigated following jaw surgery, because she began producing more than 1000 g of stools per day in contrast to the normal stool weight of less than 100 g. No abnormalities were detected on a range of gastrointestinal tests, so the woman was discharged. Following tests and complications requiring intervention in another medical center, she then returned to Baylor for further examination having suffered 3 years of excessive diarrhea. She denied any use of laxatives or diuretics when asked, but subsequent chromatographic testing of her urine revealed that she was taking bisacodyl, a well-known laxative. On confronting her and her husband, she denied knowledge of bisacodyl, but her husband eventually found an empty packet of laxatives hidden in her closet. Further questioning then revealed that the onset of diarrhea had occurred shortly after the woman had been shown to be infertile and unable to have children. She had also over the years had a number of seemingly unnecessary surgical operations, such as for jaw correction and tooth grinding, and she had obtained employment in a doctor's surgery where she had improved her knowledge of medicine. However, following her interviews at Baylor she subsequently refused to be interviewed by any more psychiatrists, only by doctors from other medical specialties.

The diagnostic systems such as DSM are careful to distinguish the factitious disorders from so-called malingering in that malingering involves the feigning of illness or disease for financial or other obvious gain. However, while the factitious presentation might not be motivated by financial or similar gain the periods of professional medical attention, plus associated care from friends and family around these medical difficulties and procedures, do seem to provide sufficient motivation to help us understand the disorders. Of course, because of the deceptive nature of the presentation of problems to others, these patients present an extremely difficult and challenging group with whom to carry out any form of research.

Abuse

Earlier in this chapter we considered how factors such as temperament, attachment, and parenting style can impact on the development of socio-emotional functioning. Implicit in the discussion of these topics and in subsequent sections was the problem of child abuse and the consequences of such abuse for the child's development and possible psychopathology.

The issue of child abuse has a long and complex history, and historically what may have been deemed as normal practice would often now be seen as abusive. For example, child labor was widely practiced in Victorian Britain, though a series of Factory Acts first restricted child labor to those aged 9 years and above, then to a maximum of 12 hours per day up to 60 hours per week. Children were employed in a wide range of work including agriculture, mining, domestic employment, and factories. In the present day, most developed countries have very low rates of child labor, but developing countries such as in Africa and Asia still have very high rates. The UNICEF website (<http://data.unicef.org/child-protection/child-labour>, accessed September 18, 2013) shows the percentage of children aged 5–14 years engaged in child labor worldwide. For example, an estimated 34% of children in Ghana and an estimated 41% of children in Zambia are engaged in child labor; the figures show that only a small proportion of these live in urban areas and the majority of child labor occurs in rural agriculture with parents as the employers.

A second example of how things have changed across time is the use of physical punishment for children, especially in the developed world. In Roman times, the law permitted the father of a child to carry out any form of physical punishment, including killing the child. Corporal punishment was widely used until recent times in almost all home and school settings, with Sweden being the first country to ban corporal punishment in 1979 because it was seen as being abusive to the child. The UN figures suggest that domestic corporal punishment has now been banned in 32 different countries worldwide.

The point to draw from these preliminary remarks is that the definition of child abuse raises a number of issues and problems because of the diversity of cultural practices, especially across historical time. Nevertheless, there is now general agreement among researchers and others that child abuse can be usefully divided into at least four different types (e.g., Finkelhor, 2008):

1. Childhood neglect—the failure of a caregiver to provide basic needs for the well-being of a child, such as food, clothing, shelter, or other types of care, that put the child's health at risk. Finkelhor's summaries of US data on child maltreatment showed that most child abuse takes the form of neglect, with an estimate that about 80% of cases fall into this category. There can be serious long-term consequences for the sufferers of neglect, including physical and mental health problems, and later difficulties in socio-emotional functioning which lead to difficulties in establishing and maintaining relationships.

2. Physical abuse—any form of physical aggression directed at a child by an adult, including beatings, punching, slapping, burning, or hitting. As noted above, the use of corporal punishment both in the home and in schools has now been outlawed in many countries following proposals from the United Nations Human Rights Committee. The US data updated for 2010 (retrieved from David Finkelhor's summary at <http://www.unh.edu/ccrc/>, accessed September 21, 2013) showed that there were 118,700 substantiated cases of childhood physical abuse in the USA in 2010, a rate of 16.2 per 10,000. In 2010 there were 1529 confirmed cases in the USA in which physical abuse led to the death of the child.

3. Emotional/psychological abuse—examples include excessive criticism, humiliation, withholding communication, denigration, or other ways of psychologically undermining the child's capacities, well-being, and relationships. In some ways this is the most difficult type of abuse to define and measure because of the sometimes subtle nature of the attacks on the child, but the consequences include delays in development, problems in socio-emotional functioning, and later risk of psychopathology.

4. Sexual abuse—abuse of a child by an adult for the purposes of sexual gratification that can include a range of activities such as sexual touching, exposure of sexual parts, use of a child in making pornographic material, and pressurizing a child into sexual activities. David Finkelhor's updated data for the USA show that in 2010 there were 63,300 cases of sexual abuse confirmed by the various children's authorities, that is a rate of 8.6 per 10,000. However, Finkelhor does note that there has been a long-term decline of 62% in rates of sexual abuse in the USA from 1990 to 2010.

These four categories of abuse are the major types that are now considered in studies of childhood development. However, as we noted above, there are other issues such as child labor where questions of abuse can arise, but with the proviso of vastly different cultural practices, for example in relation to the widespread use of child labor in agricultural communities in many parts of the world. A further type of child abuse, but one that is usually only considered with the addiction problems, is when a woman continues to use drugs or alcohol throughout pregnancy, thereby leading to teratogenic problems in the child such as in fetal alcohol syndrome and related disorders. Fetal alcohol syndrome occurs when a woman continues to use high levels of alcohol during pregnancy. Alcohol crosses the placental barrier and causes damage to the developing nervous system of the fetus; the baby is often premature with a low birthweight. In the USA and Europe it is estimated that up to 2 per 1000 births are affected by the syndrome (e.g., Abel and Sokol, 1987), making it one of the leading causes of intellectual disability at birth.

One of the problems with studying the long-term effects of childhood abuse is that typically multiple forms of abuse may be experienced by the same child, such that a child who is sexually abused may also be physically and emotionally abused as well; this can make it very hard to disentangle specific effects of different types of abuse (Finkelhor, 2008). Much research has examined the effects of abuse retrospectively, for example through interviews with people who have already developed certain types of disorders later in life. Rates of abuse seem to be elevated in most of the various psychiatric diagnoses. For example, Van Egmond and Jonker (1988) found that 52% of people self-harming for the first time and 77% of repeat cases had experienced either physical or sexual abuse in childhood. High rates of physical and sexual abuse are reported in the dissociative disorders, especially where these are associated with identity problems (e.g., Ross et al., 1990). In the area of psychosis, a review of a number of relevant studies reported rates of physical and sexual abuse in women with psychosis ranging from 51 to 97% (Goodman et al., 1997). Mueser et al. (1998) further reported that although they found high rates of childhood sexual abuse in adult women with psychosis, in many cases there were retraumatizing sexually abusive experiences in adulthood. Elevated rates of abuse have also been reported in the eating disorders, anxiety disorders, unipolar depression, and bipolar disorders (e.g., Hyun et al., 2000). In summary, although the mechanisms and the effects are still poorly understood, the experience of one or more forms of childhood abuse puts the individual at increased risk of a wide range of physical and psychological problems later in life.

Summary of Social Drive Disorders

In this chapter we have considered the most diverse set of conditions of any of the chapters in this book. The problems have ranged across difficult temperament, problems in attachment, different styles of parenting, neurodevelopmental disorders such as ASD, factitious disorders, and the possible consequences of child abuse. The sheer diversity of the range of biological and psychosocial factors and their possible interactions have only recently begun to be researched, with areas such as that of autism beginning to offer intriguing insights into the range of factors that can impact on socio-emotional functioning.

Table 5.5 gives a preliminary sketch of how this diverse range of factors might interact to produce disorders in socio-emotional functioning (note that *acquired loss* of socio-emotional functioning by reason of disease or injury will be considered in

Table 5.5: Drive–emotion–cognition analysis of social drives.

Drive	Emotion	Cognition
Social drives	↑Social-emotional functioning	↑ Executive functioning
Gene–environment (e.g., temperament–attachment)	↓ Social-emotional functioning	↓ Executive functioning

Chapter 7). The social drives have been summarized into a set of gene–environment interactions, because except in some very extreme cases where the genetic damage may be very severe the outcomes of different genetic starting points may be either positive or negative according to a range of environmental factors that interact with them. For example, so-called difficult temperaments can be more advantageous in certain environments in which easy temperaments might be a disadvantage. Equally, some attachment problems and parenting styles may impact on easy temperaments to lead to problematic developmental outcomes, whereas, as shown in Table 5.5, the right attachment pattern and parenting style can lead to superior socio-emotional functioning. The table also summarizes the impact on cognition under the general heading of executive functions, but these are meant in the widest possible sense and will also be returned to in Chapter 7 when disorders of cognition are considered in more detail. The important point, as we stressed in the discussion of ASD, is that high-level socio-emotional capacities such as TOM and empathy require a set of underlying basic cognitive processes like holistic face perception, cross-modal perceptual integration, and language and communication skills, the absence of any of which could lead to problems in the high-level socio-emotional skills.

Conclusions

In this chapter rather than conceptualizing the social drive disorders within the DEC framework we have drawn attention to a diverse range of factors, including temperament, attachment, parenting, personality disorders, neurodevelopmental disorders, factitious disorders, and childhood abuse, that could lead to such disorders. How some or all of these factors might interact to lead to disorders or problems with socio-emotional functioning has only just begun to be explored and could occupy researchers in psychology and allied disciplines for at least the next 100 years or so if we are to begin to understand the complex interactions involved. As humans, we are a social species and our most sophisticated high-level social skills have developed in order to facilitate and help us understand our interactions with our fellows. Indeed, it is possible that consciousness itself may have developed at least in part because of our need to optimize our social interactions through an understanding of how both our own and other's minds might work (see, e.g., Humphrey, 2008). At the moment we know so little, and what bits of research there are tend to be carried out in isolation; however, as these areas begin to talk to each other the future should hold exciting discoveries about exactly how these factors interact to produce high social functioning or problematic social functioning.

DISORDERS OF EMOTIONS

In a completely sane world madness is the only freedom

J. G. Ballard

Introduction

This chapter is primarily based on more detailed accounts that we have presented elsewhere (see Power and Dalgleish, 2008; Power, 2010) of how the five basic emotions of anxiety, sadness, anger, disgust, and happiness can be put together to provide a theoretical basis for the understanding of a range of emotional features including complex emotions, culture-specific emotions, emotion regulation, and the emotion disorders. The present account therefore draws heavily from previous work, though it will be fitted into the DEC framework that we have argued in previous chapters needs to be used in order to understand psychological disorders. Before turning our attention to a consideration of the emotion disorders we will therefore begin with a short recap of what the five basic emotions are and how complex emotions are derived from them. Chapter 3 also presented an overview of some of these ideas about basic emotions, which we will expand upon here.

Basic Emotions

The world's leading emotion researcher, Paul Ekman, tells a very interesting story about how he became convinced that there is a set of basic emotions that are universally recognizable in all cultures. Ekman (2003) recounts how as a young scientist he assumed, like most researchers in anthropology and psychology in the 1960s, that emotions and emotion expression were primarily culture-specific, and he dismissed the suggestion of Darwin (1872) that there might be universals in emotion and facial expression to such an extent that:

> I was so convinced that he [Darwin] was wrong that I didn't bother to read his book (Ekman, 2003, p. 2).

At this time Ekman received a grant which allowed him to test the universality versus culture-specific hypothesis in a range of cultures including the Fore in the highlands of Papua and New Guinea, who had been completely isolated from the modern world and had no television, photography, or written language. Again, Ekman is worth quoting directly:

> Are expressions universal, or are they, like language, specific to each culture? Irresistible! I really didn't care who proved to be correct, although I didn't think it would be [universality] . . . I found just the opposite of what I thought I would discover (Ekman, 2003, p. 3).

To cut a long story short, Ekman found, both to his and other researchers' surprise, evidence for the universality of facial expression of emotion across a wide range of different cultures.

In subsequent years, Ekman has at various times proposed different lists of basic emotions, initially considering the six emotions of fear, anger, surprise, disgust, happiness, and sadness to be basic, but then adding contempt as a seventh. However, more recently he has divided happiness up into sensory pleasure (which Ekman suggests could be five emotions rather than one), plus amusement, contentment, excitement, relief, wonderment, ecstasy, fiero (a type of pride), naches (another type of pride), elevation, gratitude, and schadenfreude (Ekman, 2003). These developments illustrate both the great strengths and the fatal flaws in Ekman's approach to emotion. Ekman has primarily based his approach to emotion on a single system, the face, with occasional dips into the body's peripheral psychophysiology. Unfortunately, at no point has he ever presented a full definition of emotion, otherwise sensory pleasures such as the taste of food would not be categorized as an emotion; emotions such as contempt would be analyzed as complex rather than basic emotions (Power and Dalgleish, 2008); and reactions such as surprise and startle would be seen as part of an orienting response but not as emotions in themselves. Part of the problem is that Ekman rejects appraisal as a necessary feature of emotion; thus, in his inclusion of sensory pleasures as emotions he argues explicitly that these happen too fast for appraisal processes therefore appraisal cannot be an essential part of emotion. But hang on a minute! That sounds the wrong way round to us; what if appraisal processes are precisely what differentiates emotion from non-emotion states? And, moreover, what if appraisal processes can also become fast and automated if, for example, there are oft-repeated sequences? For instance, what if every time a child cried or was miserable his mother gave him chocolate to cheer him up? The taste of chocolate may then come to be appraised in an emotionally positive way, though this appraisal process may become fast and automatic. However, the crucial distinction here is that a particular taste comes to generate emotion automatically via the associative route in SPAARS, but only this particular taste has such an emotional effect—other tastes, despite occurring very rapidly, would still not have an inherent emotional evaluation.

In order to understand some of the problems that have arisen in emotion theory and research, we suggest therefore that too many even eminent researchers have over-focused on one system at the expense of others. While Ekman has over-focused on facial expression, others such as Davidson (e.g., Davidson, 2000) and Russell (e.g., Russell, 1994), who have offered dimensional approaches to emotion (see Power and Dalgleish, 2008), have over-focused on conscious affect at the expense of other systems. However, the emotion system is based on multiple systems that have functions other than just the processing or the expression of emotion. For example, the face has multiple social expressive and communication functions that not only involve emotion—expressions of welcome, surprise, startle, understanding, puzzlement, pain, or whatever; conscious affect is experienced in relation to a whole variety of events, situations, and internal and external systems—pain, hunger, thirst, sexual excitement, and temperature are just a few examples of the many affects and blends of affects that can occur but which are not inherently emotional. In order to help us through this labyrinth, let us return to the guiding thread that we believe the SPAARS model offers in relation to basic emotions and their number and function.

SPAARS and Basic Emotions

The basic emotions that have been most widely agreed upon and included in almost all modern lists are the five shown in Table 6.1. That is, almost all commentators would agree that the emotions of anger, sadness, fear, disgust, and happiness are "basic" according to a range of criteria, though we have drawn the list from the seminal work of Oatley and Johnson-Laird (1987). Ekman (e.g., Ekman, 1999) has done most to summarize what the criteria of "basicness" are, and these criteria include the universality of the emotion, its association with specific signals (e.g., particular facial expressions), its presumed innateness, its early appearance during child development, its fast and automatic generation, and a typically fast pattern of recovery. These characteristics do of course begin to change during development with the pressures of culture and family that shape the regulation and expression of different emotions according to local "display rules." In addition, more complex emotions develop with time, some of which may be unique to a culture but whose starting point is one or more of the basic emotions from which they are therefore derivable (cf. Johnson-Laird and Oatley, 1989).

We have argued elsewhere (see Power and Dalgleish, 1997, 2008) that the essential defining aspect differentiating one emotion from another is its core appraisal, and we have offered a set of core appraisals in Table 6.1. These core appraisals are based on

Table 6.1: Five basic emotions.

Basic emotion	Appraisal
Sadness	Loss or failure (actual or possible) of a valued role or goal
Happiness	Successful move toward or completion of a valued role or goal
Anger	Blocking or frustration of a role or goal through a perceived agent
Fear	Physical or social threat to self or a valued role or goal
Disgust	Elimination or distancing from a person, object, or idea repulsive to the self, and to valued roles and goals

a set of relevant goals and plans for the individual, so let us consider briefly each of the five basic emotions. Each appraisal refers to a goal-based juncture, in which the goals are personally relevant whether in an immediate and direct manner or in a more indirect, abstract, or aesthetic way.

Sadness is a consequence of the appraisal that there is an actual loss, or a possible loss, of a valued role or goal; thus, losses of key significant others involve the loss of that relationship together with a range of subsidiary goals and plans that are entailed in key relationships. Equally, sadness could result from the loss of a favorite pen, or the memory of the loss of childhood, or the imagined loss of our job, or that someone important to us such as a child or our favorite team failed to achieve something that we had hoped for. The losses therefore can be real or imagined, they can affect us directly or indirectly because they happen to other people that are important to us, they can be recalled from our own past or can be experienced empathically or aesthetically when losses happen in a film or a novel to someone that we have identified with.

In contrast to sadness, *happiness* refers to the appraisal of movement toward or completion of a valued role or goal. In this definition, we restrict "happiness" to brief states such as joy or elation rather than the state of "life satisfaction" or Aristotle's notion of *eudaimonea* to which the highly overworked English word "happiness" also refers (see Power, in press). These brief states of happiness occur when we complete something, or win something, or do a good day's work, or get to meet someone we like, or our child does well in her homework, or our football team wins a game, or the right person gets voted in as Prime Minister, or we recall a success that we had at school. At this point, it is worth returning briefly to Ekman's (2003) confusion about positive emotion states in his claim that states such as amusement, gratitude, and schadenfreude should also be given the status of basic emotions. We dispute such an approach and argue that each of these emotions is derivable from the basic emotion of happiness, as we have defined it here, as follows. *Amusement* is typically an aesthetic emotion, the equivalent of sadness or fear experienced at the movies—so let us use this as an excuse to tell a risqué tale and see why it (hopefully) evokes (some) amusement:

> A young woman was sitting on a very crowded bus when a frail old lady got on and stood right in front of her. The young woman, however, didn't stand up to offer the old woman a seat, even though it was normal and expected to do so. Eventually the old woman said to her "I am sorry, my dear, but would you mind giving me your seat, because I am too old to stand up?" "Oh, I am so sorry," replies the young woman, "but you see I am pregnant and I have been told I should not exert myself so I need to stay sitting down." "My dear, I really do apologize. I had no idea you were pregnant, because, you know, it really doesn't show." "No," comes the reply "you are right! It really doesn't show after two hours, does it!"

An amusing story typically creates a hypothetical scenario with a set of expectations that are not fulfilled for an unexpected reason. In the story quoted, an expected action does not occur (the old woman is not offered the seat) for an unexpected but joyful reason (the young woman is allegedly pregnant), though the apparently joyful reason has again an unexpected element to it because it refers to a wished-for goal rather than one that has actually been achieved. Of course, one should not labor such analyses of humor (please excuse the bad pun), but indirect or empathic involvement in such fictional scenarios provides a range of brief emotion states that the makers of soap operas rely on for their success.

The third basic emotion that we consider in Table 6.1 is *anger*. The key appraisal that we and others have proposed for the generation of anger is the blocking of a goal, plan, or role through a perceived agent. For example, you are at work and are behind with a grant application deadline, you go to the photocopier and there are two people there chatting away and in no hurry to finish with the photocopier. You feel your irritation increasing and eventually feel quite angry. By their actions they are blocking the completion of your goal; even though they are unaware of this goal, by their agency they are preventing you completing it. This example highlights why even *inanimate* objects can be appraised as agents which are deliberately blocking our goal completion. The next time you go to the photocopier with only minutes to the grant application deadline, you find that it has broken down and you kick out at it in anger and frustration. We *know* that inanimate objects like photocopiers, computers, and that cupboard at home that will never open properly all deliberately set out to make our lives problematic!

At this point, it is also worth noting some issues raised by the earlier *non-appraisal* theories of anger. One of the most influential of these theories has been Leonard Berkowitz's (e.g., Berkowitz, 1999) frustration–aggression hypothesis. Berkowitz has argued that there are a number of drives or states that make people more aggressive. For example, if people are too hot, if they are in pain, if they are thirsty, or in some other state of discomfort, Berkowitz and others have amassed a considerable body of evidence to show that anger, frustration, and aggression are much more likely to occur. However, as DiGiuseppe and Tafrate (2007) have argued, this body of data can also be taken as evidence for the automatic route to emotion generation within the SPAARS model. In a similar way to how we can get angry with photocopiers and recalcitrant cupboards so we can also get angry with states of the personal environment (too hot, too windy, too humid, or whatever) and states of our bodies (too hot, too sweaty, or whatever). There is no question that such reactions can occur without deliberate conscious appraisal via the automatic route, but even here these reactions are modifiable because of conscious appraisals. To recall our example from Chapter 3, if you have paid thousands of dollars to travel to a hot country for your summer vacation you are more likely to feel pleasure while lying on the beach all hot and sweaty than anger and frustration—the context and meaning of the situation are crucially important, not simply the temperature of the body.

The fourth basic emotion in Table 6.1 is *fear* or *anxiety*. The primary level at which fear is generated is at the appraisal of *physical* threat to the physical body; thus, the bear charging at you through the woods makes you so terrified that you climb a tree faster than you ever thought you could. Unfortunately, though, it turns out to be a rare species of tree-climbing bear that was chasing you. . . . Alternatively, your boss has asked to see you. You know that you have been under-performing at work and rumors have been going round that the company has not been doing well and that cuts are going to be made. In this case, your *physical* self is not in any direct danger, but your *social* self and your valued work roles and goals are under threat. The night before your meeting you cannot sleep at all because of anxiety about the meeting with your boss in the morning. In the third example of anxiety, it is someone important to you rather than you yourself that is the source of the anxiety. Your child has just been taken into hospital for emergency investigations of abdominal pains of unknown cause. You feel so anxious and worried that you are unable to work or think about anything other than your child's well-being and what the outcome might be. In fact, this example relates to recent classifications of the etiological trauma for the development of PTSD; thus, DSM, as we saw in Chapter 2, includes traumatic events that happen to people who are significant to us such as parents, partners, and children and not just traumatic events that happen to ourselves.

These examples of the appraisal of anxiety all share in common a threat to something that is important or valuable to us—whether it is our physical existence, our social standing, or our key relationships. The function of anxiety in these different circumstances is to motivate us to change something in order to protect what is valuable to us. These protective or defensive actions can take of the order of milliseconds as we jump away from a speeding car or can be of a much more long-term nature when we give our children vitamin supplements because we are worried about their future health, or we switch to unleaded petrol because of our worries about the environment.

The fifth and final basic emotion listed in Table 6.1 is that of *disgust*. The origins of disgust in reactions to food and bodily products have been commented on since at least the time of Darwin (Rozin and Fallon, 1987). This primary focus on food led some earlier theorists to define the key appraisal for disgust around gustatory goals (Oatley and Johnson-Laird, 1987), but we have argued against this narrow view of the emotion of disgust, given that even in relation to bodily products there are many non-food related things that can evoke disgust, including phlegm and sexual bodily products (Power and Dalgleish, 2008). Interestingly, the only bodily products that do not seem to evoke disgust are tears, which is probably because tears are uniquely human—no other animal sheds tears as part of emotion expression and therefore tears are perceived as the least "animal-like" of all bodily products (Power, 1999). While we acknowledge the importance of disgust in food and food-waste products, we nevertheless prefer to consider the relevant appraisal in terms of a more general repulsion toward any object, person, or idea that is seen as distasteful to the self and significant others.

The disgust-based reactions that are seen in some of the eating disorders in which food or certain foodstuffs and aspects of body shape and size become repulsive seem relatively straightforward, and we will not discuss them here as they were considered in detail in Chapter 4. Perhaps less obvious is the role we suggest that disgust plays in depression, and in some types of phobias, OCD, and PTSD, as we will expand upon later in this chapter. In all of these examples, there is some aspect of the self or the world that is seen as unwanted and contaminating; thus in OCD it may be certain aspects of the world that are seen as dirty or contaminating, whereas in depression it is part of the self that becomes unwanted and loathsome and that the person tries to get rid of. We will of course be considering these examples in detail.

In summary, we believe that these five basic emotions of sadness, happiness, anger, anxiety, and disgust provide the building blocks for our emotional lives and therefore for the full range of emotional disorders that are encountered. Before we look at these disorders in more detail, however, it is necessary to consider two further aspects of this approach to emotion: first, the idea that all other emotions are derived from one or more basic emotions; and, secondly, the related proposal that emotions can become "coupled" with each other in ways that can be detrimental and form the basis of some of the emotional disorders.

Complex Emotions

One of the central tenets of the basic emotions approach is that all complex emotions are derived from the set of five basic emotions. These derivations can either occur through additional cognitive elaboration of one basic emotion, through the blending together of different basic emotions, or through the process of coupling mentioned earlier. Examples of cognitive elaboration shown in Table 6.2 would include worry as an elaboration of fear in which there is rumination about the future, and guilt as a form of disgust that is directed toward an action carried out by the self. Examples of emotion blends include contempt and nostalgia; thus, contempt, although listed under anger in Table 6.2, typically includes a measure of disgust combined with anger directed toward the person or object of contempt. Similarly, nostalgia, although listed under happiness, also includes a measure of sadness directed toward the person or situation that is the object of the nostalgia. Table 6.2 also illustrates another feature of the complexity of emotions, which is that in everyday usage the same emotion term

Table 6.2: Complex emotions.

Basic emotion	Examples of complex emotions
Fear	Embarrassment (1)
	Worry
Sadness	Grief
Anger	Envy
	Jealousy
	Contempt
Happiness	Joy
	Love
	Nostalgia
Disgust	Guilt
	Shame
	Embarrassment (2)

can come to represent different emotion states. Thus, Table 6.2 illustrates the case of embarrassment, one form of which is primarily derived from fear (e.g., a negative social evaluation anxiety), the second of which is derivable from disgust (e.g., a mild version of shame), and at least one further version (not shown) which is a positive version (e.g., when being complimented in public). Another example of multiple uses of the same word in everyday language is the word "disgust" itself, which in addition to referring in everyday language to a state of repulsion is also used to refer to being angry as in "I am disgusted with you for turning up late" (Power, 2006). The third category, that of coupling, follows similar lines to the ideas of cognitive elaboration and blending, but we will consider it separately in the next section on Emotion Coupling because of its putative role in psychopathology.

The second feature that should be noted about this approach to basic and derived complex emotions can be illustrated by analogy to language. Language is also based on a limited number of symbols such as letters, words, or ideographs, but from these an infinite number of different combinations can be generated. Similarly, three primary colors can be combined to give an infinite number of hues, tones, and blends. So, although five might not sound like a large number to begin with, once you have allowed for the range of subtle personal, interpersonal, and cultural elaborations, and the infinite number of potential blends of two or more basic emotions, then the emotion system has the potential to generate a myriad of unique as well as universal emotion states. There is no question that both historically and cross-culturally certain unique emotions have been apparent; classic examples of these unique emotions include the medieval state of "awe," a religious emotion felt in the presence of God, and the state of "accidie" which was experienced as a type of spiritual fatigue (Harre, 1987; Oatley, 2004). There are also a range of "culture-bound syndromes" that clearly incorporate some unique emotion and belief states. For example, *koro* is a condition in Southeast Asian men in which those affected experience feelings of their penis shrinking back into their body, typically accompanied by much anxiety and distress (see Chapter 2).

Emotion Coupling

One of the proposals that we made in developing the SPAARS approach to emotion was that certain emotion modules might become "coupled" with each other in ways that might lead to psychopathology (Power and Dalgleish, 1997, 2008) (see Chapter 3). There have been one or two related ideas in the psychopathology literature, such as in the influential ideas of "fear of fear" (e.g., Goldstein and Chambless, 1978) and similar ideas about "depression about depression." The "fear of fear" idea is especially relevant for understanding how someone who has experienced an extremely aversive state such as a panic attack might go to considerable efforts to avoid such an experience in the future; that is, they might successfully avoid having a further panic attack through continued avoidance, but nevertheless live in a state of anxiety. We believe that similar couplings occur not just within emotion categories, as in these examples, but can also occur between emotion categories, and that these couplings are often linked to psychopathology, as shown in Table 6.3.

Examples of "coupled" emotions shown in Table 6.3 include: happiness–anxiety and happiness–anger, both of which are sometimes seen in manic states; anxiety–disgust seen in some phobias, OCD, and types of PTSD; sadness–disgust seen in depression; and sadness–anger seen in grief (see Power and Dalgleish, 2008). Each of the examples in any individual case is more complex than merely consisting of coupling, as will be shown later. Nevertheless, they provide examples of different types of coupling mechanisms. For example, in PTSD the victim may evaluate his experience of anxiety in a rejecting self-disgust fashion, which can happen to some male victims of assault who had seen themselves as tough and invulnerable prior to the assault; their feelings of panic and anxiety are now appraised as weak and pathetic and they lead to feelings of self-disgust as well as anxiety. In this PTSD example, the coupling is caused by the appraisal of one emotion as weak and unacceptable, thereby leading to a second emotion. Again, in depression the coupling of self-disgust can occur directly to the feelings of sadness, especially in some depressions in men, but more typically the feelings of self-disgust are directed at the self in addition to any specific emotions. For example, following the break-up of a love relationship a woman might feel sadness because of the loss and be anxious about how she will survive alone, while at the same time despising herself for needing a relationship and not being completely self-sufficient. In such cases, the coupling may be both direct and indirect in that it is more the cause of the sadness (needing a relationship)

Table 6.3: Examples of coupled emotions in problematic emotion states.

	Anger	Anxiety	Sadness	Disgust	Happiness
Anger		PTSD-1	Grief	Bulimia	Mania-1
Anxiety		Fear of fear Phobias-1 OCD-1	Depression-2 PTSD-2	Phobias-2 OCD-2 PTSD-3	Mania-2
Sadness				Depression-1	Mania-3
Disgust					Mania-4
Happiness					

than perhaps the sadness itself that becomes the focus of the self-disgust (Power and Tarsia, 2007).

The proposal for the coupling of emotions as suggested in the SPAARS model has primarily been supported by clinical and anecdotal evidence. Recently, however, one of my PhD students, John Fox, worked with a group of students with bulimia in a priming paradigm to test the prediction that anger and disgust could be coupled in bulimia (Fox and Harrison, 2008). A group of female students who met clinical criteria for bulimia together with a matched healthy control group were both given an anger induction task. Their levels of anger and disgust were tested immediately before and immediately after the anger induction procedure. The results showed that both groups had similar levels of disgust and anger before the priming procedure, and that afterwards both demonstrated significant increases in anger (though somewhat more in the bulimia group); most interesting, however, was the finding of a significant increase in the levels of disgust in the bulimia group but no change in the control group. John Fox has now replicated and extended these findings to a group of participants with clinical eating disorders (Fox et al., 2013). These results show support for the proposed coupling of anger and disgust in bulimia, and also how the priming methodology can be used to test predicted couplings in other disorders, in addition to the self-report methods that we have also used (Power and Tarsia, 2007). However, without further ado, we will now examine emotion disorders linked to each of the basic emotions, beginning with anger.

Anger Disorders

We have discussed previously the idea that anger disorders can arise because an individual might feel too little anger, in addition to the more common presentation of too much anger (Power, 2010). Although such experiences are theoretically interesting, and in some cases can be regarded as pathological, especially if they lead to rare but excessively violent outbursts, the essence of the so-called anger disorders is really about too much anger or anger that is inappropriate (DiGiuseppe and Tafrate, 2007). In this section we consider these reactions and also the case of morbid jealousy. For each of the five basic emotions we will first consider possible emotion disorders that primarily involve the emotion itself, disorders that may be based on complex emotions derived from the basic emotion, before we consider ways in which the emotion might couple with one or more other basic emotions as illustrated in Table 6.3.

Table 6.4: Drive–emotion–cognition (DEC) analysis of anger disorders.

Drive	Emotion	Cognition
Survival drives Dominance	(Basic) Anger	Blocking Thwarting Insult Non-normative models of self
Sex	(Complex) Jealousy	Trust Infidelity
Survival	(Coupled) Anger–anxiety Anger–sadness	Threat Loss

The DEC starting point for the analysis of possible anger disorders is presented in Table 6.4. Although threats to survival—whether this involves physical or social survival—can be appraised to lead to anxiety (see the section Anxiety Disorders), they can also lead to anger. The basic appraisal in anger (namely the blocking of a goal by a perceived agent; see Table 6.1) can refer to the basic goals connected to physical or social survival, a possibility that has traditionally been captured by the well-known "fight-or-flight" reaction in situations of threat (e.g., Tooby and Cosmides, 1990). Anger can move from order to disorder in a number of ways. First, individuals can become angry at events in a way which most of society would regard as inappropriate. Secondly, anger can be directed at or displaced onto inappropriate agents. Thirdly, anger can be an appropriate reaction to the circumstances while being excessive in its intensity. Finally, anger can be extrinsically motivated. We will consider each of these possibilities in turn. However, the common feature of anger disorders is the excessive expression of aggression. As must be noted, excessive expressions of aggression are not invariably a consequence of anger but can also occur for other reasons and in other emotion states (e.g., see Blair et al., 2005). Aggression can also be expressed on an individual basis or by groups, as in crowd violence, with the ultimate expression of aggression being war (Power, in press). And just as wars aren't always motivated by reasons of anger or hatred but can be expressions of dominance–subordination, ideology, revenge, or whatever (e.g., Rosen, 2004), we can be clear that individual motivations behind aggression are equally varied. With that caveat in mind, we therefore now consider disorders of anger.

When the schematic models of self, world, and other differ from those that are normative, then the generation and expression of anger in an individual can appear abnormal. Averill (1982) calls this "anger gone awry." To quote:

Inappropriate behaviour, especially of a violent nature, may also result from a failure of an individual to internalise appropriate regulative rules. Of course, what is considered "appropriate" in this sense depends on the group making the valuation, namely, the dominant culture. Subgroups within the culture, whilst sharing many of the norms or values that help constitute anger, may nevertheless regulate their behaviour differently (Averill, 1982, p. 336).

A detailed discussion of the rules and regulations of such subcultures may be found in Wolfgang and Ferracuti (1967), who examine the Vendetta Barbaricina in Sardinia and the Mafia in Sicily, and in Wolfgang (1979), who has worked with populations of street boys in Philadelphia. In addition to the failure to adopt normative social rules in particular subgroups of society, there are individual differences in the makeup of the domains of knowledge of the world, self, and other. In their most extreme form such variations begin to take on clinical characteristics; for example, certain forms of paranoid personality disorder are likely to be characterized by appraisals of deliberation, avoidability, and negligence which fall outside the range of social normality. The so-called psychopath is an individual who may use combinations of reactive and instrumental aggression against others (Blair et al., 2005), who shows a failure to adopt normative rules and low affective responding.

Consider the example of Peter (taken from Power and Dalgleish, 2008):

> Peter is a 13-year-old boy with severe kidney problems which are being treated with regular and prolonged dialysis requiring frequent hospitalization. Peter gets on reasonably well with his parents and friends but has a very bad relationship with his slightly older sister, Julie. Whenever Julie is around, Peter is always bullying her and shouting at her and sometimes her very presence seems to rouse him to uncontrollable rages.

Peter may be and understandably angry at the world or fate for singling him out to have a highly disabling illness, for making him different and an object of pity. However, it seems that much of this anger is displaced onto Julie, even though it is clearly not her fault that Peter is ill. Such displacement of anger is an everyday occurrence; no doubt we have all "taken it out" on someone close or been more aggressive while driving (e.g., Lawton and Nutter, 2002). However, the displacement of anger can also become disordered and disabling to relationships and social groups.

Anger can also be directed at and displaced onto the self. An understanding of anger directed toward the self seems especially important in considering emotional order and disorder; indeed, during the earlier part of the twentieth century, self-directed anger and rage were central to a number of theories of depression, especially those from the psychoanalytic school (e.g., Freud, 1917). The pioneering work which proposed a role for self-directed anger in depression was Freud's *Mourning and Melancholia*, published in 1917 when Freud was in his 60s and had his own personal experiences of depression to draw upon. We have reviewed the limitations of Freud's ideas of the involvement in depression of anger turned inwards toward the ego in greater detail elsewhere (Power and Dalgleish, 2008), so we will spend no more time on this aspect of anger here. Nevertheless, we note the increasing interest in the possible role of anger in eating disorders (e.g., Waller et al., 2003) that we discussed in Chapter 4, and in PTSD (e.g., Novaco and Chemtob, 2002) that we will discuss later in this chapter.

A third way in which anger can become disordered is when individuals experience and express anger in ways that are entirely out of proportion to the precipitating circumstances. In these scenarios, the fact that anger is an appropriate reaction to the precipitating events and interpretations is not in question; what seems disordered is the extent and force of the individual's anger reactions. In the American television series *The Incredible Hulk* (and the later Hollywood movie directed by Ang Lee), the mild-mannered Bruce Banner often warned his would-be protagonists: "Don't make me angry, you won't like me when I'm angry." Those who foolishly ignored this warning then had to deal with a raging, towering green monster who was prepared to tear them limb from limb. While this is clearly an extreme example, we all know individuals with whom we feel the need to tip-toe around their sensibilities, fearing that the slightest provocation will elicit "Hulk-like" behavior. Some have argued that "anger attacks"—extreme examples of the inability to control one's anger—may represent a discrete clinical syndrome (e.g., Fava et al., 1993) or be a variant of bipolar disorder if there is also a history of depression (e.g., Franco, 2003). Whether or not one agrees with this proposal, there is a widespread consensus that an inability to control one's anger frequently presents as a problem in the clinic (e.g., Novaco, 1979), and this has led to the development of systematic therapeutic procedures for the development of anger control.

As we have noted, the principal problem with disproportionate, uncontrollable anger lies in the related action potentials to retaliate and aggress. A famous example from the Maudsley Hospital in London, which was the subject of a television documentary, illustrates this point:

> John [not his real name] was a man with a violent history. He had several criminal convictions for bodily harm and can recount times when he has nearly killed people in uncontrollable rages. At the time that John came into contact with mental health services he would only rarely leave his home and then he would be accompanied by several bodyguards—not to protect him from others, but to protect others from him.

In cases such as John's, it seems clear that there are few holds on the full-blown expression of anger. Such behavior seems most likely to be the result of a troubled, violent development in which anger and aggression are socialized as appropriate and acceptable responses to events, or can reflect the loss of inhibitory control from neurological damage if it appears later in life (e.g., Blair et al., 2005).

In terms of complex emotions that derive from the basic emotion of anger, disorders of jealousy are worth some comment. Examples of pathological jealousy are common in the cinema and literature. In the film *L'Enfer*, for example, Daniel Auteuil's character experiences angry, violent jealousy over his innocent and beautiful wife. In the denouement, the wife is shackled to the couple's bed while the husband stalks the room wielding a cut-throat razor. The camera shifts suddenly to the view from the window where ambulance men from the nearby psychiatric hospital can be seen approaching the house. Similarly, in Paul Sayer's novel *Howling at the Moon*, the anti-hero becomes obsessively jealous of his, again innocent, wife and, resigning his job, sets off to work each day as usual only to inhabit the house opposite from where he observes his wife's every move through binoculars, recording the details minutely. What is it that makes jealousy pathological in such cases? Clearly, the extreme nature of the different types of behavior involved is important. However, perhaps more central is the fact that in each case the jealousy is a function of beliefs which are unfounded. It is important to note that the truth value of the beliefs is not what is at issue. The belief may be a false one but understandable given the circumstances. For example, Othello's jealousy was a function of false beliefs; however, these beliefs were not unfounded as they were grounded in Iago's deception and manipulation of the situation. Interestingly, morbid jealousy is sometimes referred to as Othello syndrome, a label which, in this analysis, seems wholly unfair. A consequence of the ungrounded nature of morbid jealousy is the jealous person's attempt to provide a basis of reality to the feelings. As in *Howling at the Moon*, this can often lead to obsessive attention to the minutiae of the other's life. How can morbid jealousy be explained? The traditional Freudian view is that such unfounded jealousy is a projection of individuals' doubts about maintaining their own fidelity and ability to resist temptation. As Freud neatly summarizes "A man who doubts his own love may, or rather must, doubt every lesser thing" (Freud, 1920, p. 241). A more recent view from evolutionary psychology (e.g., Tooby and Cosmides, 1992) is that morbid sexual jealousy should be more prevalent in men in an attempt to prevent sexual infidelity in their partners, whereas morbid emotional jealousy should be more prevalent in women in an attempt to avoid resource loss which might therefore endanger survival of their children. The evidence, however, is extremely mixed and offers little support for the proposal (Harris, 2003).

Tables 6.3 and 6.4 show that the coupling of anger with other basic emotions can contribute to other types of disorders. For example, in Dalgleish and Power (2004) we argued that some types of PTSD reactions may be primarily anger based in that they can involve the coupling of anger and anxiety in reaction to the trauma. In our analysis of a series of 75 consecutive attendees at a trauma service who met the criteria for PTSD (Power and Fyvie, 2013), we found that ratings of anger were higher than ratings of anxiety in approximately 25% of cases, with additional analyses suggesting a longer and more chronic course when emotions such as anger are significantly involved in the presentation of PTSD. Additional couplings for anger that we have noted in Table 6.3 include the coupling of anger and sadness in grief, and anger and happiness in some types of mania, which we will return to in subsequent sections of this chapter.

Anxiety Disorders

Table 6.5 illustrates a range of possible disorders of anxiety, including disorders of the basic emotion, such as panic and some types of phobias, disorders of complex emotions derived from anxiety, such as worry in generalized anxiety disorder (GAD), and disorders in which anxiety is coupled with other basic emotions, as in some types of phobias, some types of OCD, and some types of PTSD. Fear and anxiety can become disordered in a variety of ways. We can experience excessive fear of relatively harmless objects or we can develop beliefs that certain things are threatening or harmful when they are not. In other situations fear or anxiety can seem appropriate but over-generalized, such as in post-traumatic reactions or chronic worry. The challenge for

Table 6.5: Drive–emotion–cognition (DEC) analysis of anxiety disorders.

Drive	Emotion	Cognition
Survival drives –Physical –Social	(Basic) Panic Anxiety	Threat
Survival drives –Physical –Social	(Complex) Jealousy	Threat Future threat
Survival drives –Physical –Social	(Coupled) Anxiety–anxiety Anxiety–anger Anxiety–sadness Anxiety–disgust Anxiety–happiness	Threat

any theory that seeks to explain both fear order and fear disorder is to account for the varieties of abnormal fear without making them seem like discrete pathological entities. Balancing this challenge is the need to integrate new ideas with the existing literature on disordered fear that is centered around the so-called anxiety disorders, while realizing that the disorders are not qualitatively different from normal fear reactions.

Within the previous DSM-IV classification system (American Psychiatric Association, 1994), the anxiety disorders were organized around the categories of phobias, PTSD, panic disorder, OCD, and GAD. However, DSM-5 (American Psychiatric Association, 2013) has extracted the OCD and PTSD categories from under the heading of anxiety disorders because of the heterogeneous nature of the emotion components in different types of OCD and PTSD, while acknowledging that anxiety is a frequent emotion in some types of OCD and PTSD. An alternative strategy, and the one taken here, is that these heterogeneous categories need to be broken up in order to reflect which of the basic emotions provides the foundation for a particular disorder. For example, we will note the existence of different types of PTSD in relation to the different basic emotions of anxiety, anger, sadness, and disgust, which indeed can sometimes present in the form of coupled basic emotions as shown in Table 6.5 (Power and Fyvie, 2013).

Some types of phobia provide clear examples of an anxiety-based disorder that is linked to physical threat, whereas examples such as social phobia and agoraphobia may be better considered as responses to social threat and relate to the social drives considered in Chapter 5. Other phobias, such as the blood–injury phobias, are more likely to be disgust-based responses, or disgust–anxiety coupled responses, so we will return to these in the later section on disgust-based disorders. Phobias are usually defined as irrational fears of objects or situations. Simple phobias involve fear of, for example, snakes or spiders combined with an ability to see that there is no reason to be afraid. Agoraphobia is somewhat different, and is characterized by fear of leaving the home or a safe environment. Agoraphobia is highly comorbid with panic problems and we will consider it briefly in the section on panic. Finally, social phobia involves anxiety about social situations and a fear of embarrassment.

We have argued elsewhere that phobic problems, particularly specific phobias, are extremely common and that in our view it is a mistake to assume that just because individuals meet the majority of criteria for a clinical diagnosis of phobia they are pathological, abnormal, or disordered in any way (Power and Dalgleish, 2008). This issue of distinguishing normal fears from phobias is a factor in epidemiological studies—community surveys nevertheless reveal that mild phobias affect an average of about 6 per 100 people, with around 2 per 1000 having a phobia that is viewed as disabling (Myers et al., 1984). Specific phobias tend to have their origins in childhood (e.g., Rutter, 1984), though a large number of childhood fears disappear as the individual matures. Social phobia and agoraphobia have a later onset (Antony and Barlow, 2002). Phobias are more usually reported by women, with estimates indicating that as many as 95% of sufferers of simple phobias are women (Rachman, 2004).

Fear-derived simple phobias are characterized by extreme fear and anxiety in the presence of the phobic stimulus, an uncontrollable desire to leave the feared situation, and, outside of the feared situation, an ability to see that the fear is unfounded. Theoretical work suggests that there are three main routes to the acquisition of such phobias (Rachman, 2004). The first is through a two-process conditioning sequence in which the phobic stimulus becomes classically conditioned to elicit fear and is then instrumentally reinforced by the subject avoiding the feared stimulus (Mowrer, 1960). The second route is through vicarious conditioning or modeling in which the individual witnesses another person's fear reaction. Finally, phobias may become acquired through the dissemination of information about the phobic object (see Field, 2006, for a discussion). Support for these three putative routes has been through simple self-report surveys (e.g., Hekmat, 1987). However, it is by no means clear that the initial emotional reactions, particularly in the vicarious route, are necessarily ones of fear. A final point is that some phobias are more common than others and this seems to reflect some form of evolutionary preparedness (Ohman and Mineka, 2001; Seligman, 1971) in which we have a propensity to quickly develop fear reactions to objects and situations that were genuinely threatening to our ancestors.

Panic was first claimed as a discrete anxiety presentation in response to the work of Klein (1981). His research in psychobiology led him to propose that panic attacks and non-panic-related anxiety are two distinct pathophysiological syndromes. Klein's work has inspired a whole body of theoretical and empirical research focusing on the idea that panic disorder originates from a genetically transmitted neurochemical abnormality which presents as a sudden surge of autonomic arousal and fear symptoms. However, later theoretical work in psychology (e.g., Clark, 1986) has suggested that such biological hypotheses represent inadequate explanations of the phenomenology of panic. Consequently, a number of psychological theories of panic have been proposed, alternatively emphasizing personality, conditioning, and information-processing analyses of the disorder. Furthermore, a considerable body of psychological research into the processes underlying panic has been carried out (see, e.g., Craske and Waters, 2005, for a review). Psychological approaches to understanding panic disorder have revolved around the idea that the panic is in some way a "fear of fear" (Goldstein and Chambless, 1978). That is, people panic because they are threatened by the presence or potential presence of fear-related phenomenal states. There are a number of variations of the fear of fear hypothesis: Pavlovian interoceptive conditioning (Goldstein and Chambless, 1978); catastrophic misinterpretation of bodily sensations (Clark, 1986); and anxiety sensitivity (McNally, 1990; Taylor, 1999). The work of David Clark has now provided the main cognitive account of panic disorder. Clark's elegantly simple model of panic owes much to the ideas of Beck (e.g., Beck, 1976). According to Clark's (1986) model of panic, "catastrophic misinter-pretations of certain bodily sensations are a necessary condition for the production of a panic attack"; thus, a panic attack may originate from the misinterpretation that an increase in heart rate is a signal for an impending heart attack, or that the onset of a slight dizzy feeling or being flushed is a sign that the individual is about to faint. Although such bodily sensations are symptoms of fear, and consequently Clark's model can be thought of as an extension of the fear of fear hypothesis, such sensa-tions are not uniquely associated with fear. So, for example, heart palpitations may result from excessive caffeine intake or exercise rather than from an interpretation or appraisal related to threat. The point, then, is that Clark's model is about the cata-strophic misinterpretation of bodily sensations whatever their cause; that is, it does not restrict itself to a fear of fear analysis (see Power and Dalgleish, 2008, for further detail and a critique).

Since its inclusion in DSM-III (American Psychiatric Association, 1980), PTSD has been the subject of a great deal of empirical and theoretical work. A number of well thought out psychological models of PTSD have been proposed, many within a cog-nitive framework (e.g., Ehlers and Clark, 2000; Foa and Rothbaum, 1998). According to DSM-IV (American Psychiatric Association, 1994), PTSD can follow traumatic events in which individuals experience a threat to their own life or the lives of others or a threat to their own or others' physical integrity. DSM-5 (American Psychiatric Association, 2013) further clarified that learning about a traumatic event happen-ing to a significant other or repeated exposure to details of traumatic events, as with emergency workers, also meet its Criterion A for PTSD diagnosis. However, although such attempts to objectively define the etiological events in PTSD are useful, we sug-gest that it is the impact of the event or events on individual's current models of self, world, and other that is central. For some this might indeed be a life-threatening car crash or a tour of duty in Vietnam; for others, however, being shouted at by their pre-viously calm and supportive boss at work might be sufficient. For DSM-IV the clinical features of PTSD following such events included:

1. Re-experiencing symptoms, such as intrusive memories, thoughts or images, and nightmares.
2. Avoidance reactions such as emotional numbing where the individual is unable to feel a range of emotions or is able to describe the trauma in a dispassionate

way, amnesia for all or part of the event, behavioral avoidance where individuals go to great lengths to avoid stimuli that will remind them of the trauma, and cognitive avoidance such as the use of distraction techniques to get rid of unwanted thoughts.

3. Arousal symptoms such as an exaggerated startle response, irritability, and hypervigilance for trauma-related information.

DSM-5 added in a fourth category of alterations to cognition and/or mood as a consequence of the trauma. In addition to anxiety, PTSD is commonly accompanied by a wide range of other emotions such as sadness, anger, guilt, and shame, which DSM-5 now lists under Criterion D4 as "fear, horror, anger, guilt, or shame." Again, we would note the importance of sadness in traumatic grief, to which we will return later. A distinctive feature in PTSD is that in many cases the intrusive memories consist of images accompanied by high levels of fear or are re-enactments of the original trauma ("flashbacks"). Herman (1992) has referred to flashbacks as "frozen memories," a term that captures their repetitive, unchanging quality. Further points about the DSM-5 revisions for PTSD include the invention of a "dissociative-type" PTSD, which has been based on very little research and which may well disappear in later editions. DSM-5 has also disappointed many trauma clinicians who find the concept of a "complex" type of PTSD, involving sustained interpersonal trauma typically experienced in childhood, to be an extremely useful clinical category, though it seems likely that the ICD-11 workgroup on PTSD may well include complex PTSD as a diagnostic category in its forthcoming ICD revision.

Generalized anxiety problems involve excessive worry about several lifestyle domains such as health, finances, relationships, and so on. Such worrying usually takes up most of the individual's time and becomes highly disabling, both for the individual concerned and for their partner, friends and family. This so-called pathological worry is associated with a number of physiological/somatic symptoms of fear or anxiety; but for diagnostic purposes it is not usually regarded as including among its domains of concern the sorts of stimuli that are associated with the other so-called anxiety disorders (e.g., a specific etiological trauma as in PTSD, the phobic object in phobias, etc.). Such generalized worry has been labeled GAD in psychiatric classification systems like the DSM. There are a variety of nosological issues involved in the conceptualization of GAD. These concern, first, the relationship between GAD, a so-called clinical disorder, and subclinical levels of chronic anxiety as measured by concepts such as trait anxiety (e.g., Spielberger et al., 1970); secondly, the relationship of GAD with depression and with mixed anxiety–depression disorders; and, thirdly, the relationship of the type of anxiety-related problems found in someone with

GAD with the type of anxiety-related problems which epitomize panic disorder. An excellent overview of the debates can be found in the book by Barlow (2002). For the purposes of the present discussion we confine ourselves to highlighting two points: first, that most individuals who meet the criteria for a diagnosis of GAD are also somewhat depressed and that this has implications for much of the research that has been carried out (Power and Dalgleish, 2008); secondly, there is clearly a relationship between subclinical chronic anxiety as measured by constructs such as trait anxiety and the clinical problem of GAD, and it does not seem unreasonable to suggest that high levels of trait-anxiety represent a vulnerability factor for the onset of GAD (e.g., Eysenck, 1997).

Obsessional states are extremely complex phenomena and may be better conceptualized as disorders of cognition, to which we will return in Chapter 7. In some ways the fear or anxiety components involved in some obsessions are the easiest aspect of the disorder to account for. Individuals might be afraid that if they do not check the gas tap then the house will blow up and people may be killed. Such anxiety is reduced by checking that the tap is switched off. What is more difficult to account for is why the obsessional individual has to check repeatedly that the gas is turned off. It is beyond the scope of this book to provide a comprehensive empirical and theoretical review of fear-based obsessional states because it does not seem clear that the emotional component is central to the disorder. Others have done this job more than adequately (e.g., Rachman, 2003; Tallis, 1995a,b). What we do wish to spend some time on, however, is the suggestion that some obsessional states can best be conceived of as disorders of disgust, particularly those involving washing compulsions and contamination-related intrusions. Until recently, the role of disgust has been sadly neglected in such cases so we present an analysis of disgust-based obsessions later in this chapter (see Disgust Disorders), but return to the general issue of OCD in Chapter 7.

Sadness Disorders

The DEC analysis of disorders of sadness is presented in Table 6.6. The basic emotion of sadness occurs on the appraisal of loss, whether the loss be temporary or permanent, directly affecting oneself or a significant other, or real or imagined (Power and Dalgleish, 2008). As with other basic emotions, the prototypical experience of sadness is relatively brief and typically lasts a matter of seconds or minutes. The disorders of sadness therefore do not just reflect the generation of sadness per se but are based on complex elaborations of the emotion and the coupling of sadness with other basic emotions, as shown in Table 6.6. The two main "disorders" of sadness are grief and

Table 6.6: Drive–emotion–cognition (DEC) analysis of sadness disorders.

Drive	Emotion	Cognition
Social drives	(Basic) Sadness	Loss
Social drives	(Complex) Grief	Loss Hopelessness
Social drives	(Coupled) Sadness–anger Sadness–self-disgust Sadness–anxiety	Loss Humiliation Hopelessness Defeat

depression, but in both cases other emotions and problematic states are invariably involved such that a "pure" disorder of sadness alone does not seem to occur.

In an attempt to understand both the lengthy nature of the normal grief reaction and the even lengthier nature of abnormal reactions, studies of the separation of children from their primary caregivers provide an important starting point. Bowlby's (1980) summary of this work showed that the child may initially go through stages of protest and despair because of the separation, but eventually, if the mother (or other primary caregiver) returns, the child may treat her as if she were a stranger. In contrast, a non-primary caregiver (perhaps the father) may be greeted with warmth and relief over the same length of separation. Bowlby's interpretation of these different reactions is that the child eventually reacts to the separation from or loss of the mother by "defensively excluding" or inhibiting his or her negative emotions. Even with the very short separations of a few minutes studied in the laboratory with the strange situation test (Ainsworth et al., 1978), a proportion of children as young as 12 months showed ambivalent positive and negative reactions to their mother's return.

A second related area from work with children focuses not so much on whether children *express* ambivalent feelings, but on whether they can *conceptualize* such ambivalence. Harter (1977, 1999), for example, noticed that many children she saw in the clinic were unable to admit to ambivalent feelings, particularly toward primary caregivers. In her subsequent work with normal children, she found that only at about 10 years of age can children acknowledge and describe these ambivalent feelings (Harter and Buddin, 1987). The following quote from Bowlby (1980) captures the same idea:

> In therapeutic work it is not uncommon to find that a person (child, adolescent or adult) maintains, consciously, a wholly favourable image of a parent, but that at a less conscious level he nurses a contrasting image in which his parent is represented as

neglectful, or rejecting, or as ill-treating him. In such persons the two images are kept apart, out of communication with each other; and any information that may be at variance with the established image is excluded (Bowlby, 1980, pp. 70–71).

This statement from Bowlby concurs remarkably with our proposals for SPAARS of two routes to emotion generation, one of which may be conscious and the other automatic, and which may lead to the generation of contrasting or conflicting emotions (Power and Dalgleish, 1999). In relation to grief, the conclusion that we draw from these findings and our previous proposals is that the loss of the main attachment figure, whether in childhood or adulthood, leads not only to the emotion of sadness but frequently also to anger at that person for abandoning the individual to an uncertain fate. However, the expression and conceptualization of such ambivalence requires a developmentally sophisticated level of maturity that many individuals may fail to negotiate or may do so only partially. Thus, the individual may feel sadness following such a loss, but feel extreme guilt about feelings of anger, or, psychologically, go one step further and idealize the lost person so that no feelings of anger could even be imaginable toward such a perfect individual. In addition, the combination of pressures on an individual in Western and other cultures to inhibit the expression of both sadness and anger following loss may all lead to the result that grief runs an atypical course (Parkes et al., 1997).

In terms of our general SPAARS model presented earlier, the experience of extreme grief consequent on the loss of an attachment figure can be seen as the impact of the loss of mutual goals, roles, and plans that the attachment figure represented. Because of the evolutionary basis of attachment, the universal experience of grief across cultures must in part have an innate foundation and must therefore involve operation of the direct access route to emotion within SPAARS. However, the effects on an individual of the loss of a significant other are so wide-ranging that multiple and continued appraisals will accompany any automatic reactions. For example, studies of the impact of bereavement in Western culture show that the nature of the impact and its consequences may differ for widows and widowers; Wortman et al. (1993) reported that widowers were particularly vulnerable to limited social relationships and problems with taking on tasks that their wives had handled, whereas widows were more vulnerable to financial strain following the death of their husbands. The net effect of these and other problems is that bereaved individuals may make appraisals that they will be unable to cope with the practical and emotional burden they have been left with. In addition, if the bereaved appraise the grief reaction itself as weak or not allowed, because of a more general rejection of negative emotions, then a more atypical course for grief may be likely. This atypical course may be more likely to occur, we would speculate, if coupling of the basic emotions of sadness and anger occurs, as shown in Table 6.6, given that many grief reactions have in addition to the primary emotion of sadness other appraisals that lead to anger. The anger may be directed at the lost individuals themselves or at others who caused the loss or did not do enough to prevent the loss; anger is more likely to occur where deaths are sudden and unexpected (e.g., Vargas et al., 1989) and may thereby explain in part why sudden and unexpected deaths may lead to more chronic or difficult grief reactions, though not always (Stroebe and Stroebe, 1993). We argued above that once such couplings of activated basic emotions occur they may reciprocally activate each other and thereby prolong the emotional state. In the case of grief, however, we must also emphasize the internal and external pressures to inhibit not only the expression of sadness but also, especially, the expression of anger toward the lost individual. The greater the attempts to inhibit one or both of the emotions of sadness and anger involved in grief, therefore, the longer the likely course of the grief reaction. The loss of the main attachment figure whether in childhood or adulthood involves nothing less than a redefinition of the self; an individual who prevents, whether consciously or unconsciously, such a process from occurring, who attempts to deny the loss of the key other, will be left with a model of the self that is maladaptive, inaccurate, and out of date (e.g., Parkes, 1993).

In summary, we propose that the experience of grief can run a number of possible courses depending on a variety of factors, the majority of which are typical and not disordered but a minority of which may become atypical in some way such that they may be labeled as "disordered." First, the cultural and familial pressures that inhibit the expression of sadness in men ("boys don't cry") and anger toward someone who has died in both men and women ("don't speak ill of the dead"). Secondly, the developmental history of the individual in which early childhood ambivalence toward the primary caregiver may have been socialized out, because the adult was, for example, unable to contain the child's anger. Thirdly, the nature of the relationship with the lost individual, that is, the degree to which the relationship was secure or ambivalent. Fourthly, the type and suddenness of the loss, for example the degree to which an individual has been able to prepare for the loss of an aging parent, versus the premature and unexpected loss of a healthy child. And, finally, the quality and the nature of the support from significant others in the individual's network ("we don't mention her name, so as not to upset him").

Depression is the classic disorder of sadness. As we noted in Chapter 1, the term melancholia was first used in the fifth century BCE by Hippocrates. Based on the ancient doctrine of the four elements, four humors were identified in blood, each of which in excess could lead to problems; thus, the melancholic type suffered an excess of black bile. Whichever type you were, though, the treatment was usually the same, namely, bloodletting. Over the subsequent thousand years or so a lot of melancholic individuals lost a lot of blood. Galen in the first century CE added further to our knowledge of melancholia, emphasizing the occurrence of, in his term, hypochondriacal symptoms in the disorder. In contrast to grief, in which we argued for the key roles of the basic emotions of sadness and anger, we suggest that depression may be derivable primarily from the basic emotions of sadness and disgust. This proposal offers an alternative to that suggested by Freud in *Mourning and Melancholia*, in which mourning was derived from sadness whereas depression was derived from sadness plus anger that was turned against the self. The key rejection of Freud's proposal for retroflective anger occurred in Bibring's (1953) classic ego psychoanalytic reanalysis of depression, a paper that anticipated all of the major cognitive approaches to the disorder (see Power and Dalgleish, 2008). Nevertheless, our proposal does hold some similarities to Freud's in that we emphasize self-condemnation and shame as defining characteristics of depression, the crucial difference being that we derive self-condemnation and shame from the basic emotion of disgust rather than from anger. We would also point out that, since Bibring's paper, most cognitive models have focused on the role of low self-esteem in depression; thus, in both Beck's (1976) cognitive therapy and in Abramson et al.'s (1978) learned helplessness reformulation the self is seen as culpable for negative events, and is considered to be worthless, failed, or bad. All of these aspects of the self can be derived from the turning of the basic emotion of disgust against the self, especially in shame, such that aspects of the self are seen as bad and have to be eliminated or rejected from the self.

Another basic emotion that is frequently observed along with depression is that of anxiety; thus, self-report measures of depression and anxiety typically correlate at about 0.7 across a range of populations (Goldberg and Goodyer, 2005). Indeed, the so-called tripartite model proposed by Clark and Watson (1991) and Clark (2000) argues that there is a common core of "negative affect" that forms the major component of a range of emotions including depression and anxiety. While there is much to be commended in such analyses, we take issue with the basic underlying model: first, because so-called negative affects are not necessarily experienced as negative, as we have argued previously; secondly, because most of the results are based on student populations or, even in their tests of the model, patient groups such as those with drug problems that do not directly test the model (Watson et al., 1995a,b); and, thirdly, because individuals may show *less* anxiety rather than more as they become increasingly depressed (Peterson et al., 1993). These points do not in any way deny the high comorbidity of depression and anxiety, particularly for less severe depression, and, indeed, there is every likelihood that the coupling together of the basic emotions involved in depression together with anxiety will undoubtedly lead to a prolongation of this distressing state. The proposal, however, is that anxiety is not a defining feature of depression, nor depression of anxiety. What we do wish to emphasize is that severe life events often unfold over time rather than occur suddenly and out of the blue, and they often occur in the context of long-term related difficulties (e.g., Brown et al., 1995). In addition, the threat of loss may subsequently turn into an actual loss (Finlay-Jones and Brown, 1981), and so a state of anxiety in which the individual remains hopeful may turn into a state of depression in which the individual feels hopeless (Alloy et al., 2006).

The key coupling of the basic emotions of sadness and disgust that we argue is the basis of some presentations of depression is shown in Table 6.6. So why have we given disgust such a central role? We offer a number of reasons for this, some of which are more speculative than others, though we accept that the overall proposal requires additional empirical testing. Nevertheless, we are persuaded by ideas from a number of different areas that the role of disgust has largely been unrecognized in the development of emotional and other disorders. Evidence that shame and humiliation may be important factors in the onset of depression has come from two separate studies of the same population in Islington, north London. In the first study, Brown et al. (1995) reported that life events that lead to feelings of humiliation and entrapment in addition to loss or danger were more predictive of onset of depression than loss or danger events that did not include humiliation and entrapment. In the second study, Andrews (1995) found that a strong link between childhood physical and sexual abuse and the later occurrence of depression was mediated by the experience of bodily shame which typically developed in the teenage years, presumably in response to the teenager's own physical and sexual development. Andrews interpreted her findings as evidence for Gilbert's (1989) proposal that shame relates to the experience of defeat and inferiority, implicit in the experience of abuse (see Gilbert, 2004, for a summary). A further replication of the Islington studies was carried out by Kendler et al. (2003) using a large twin register in Virginia; they found that loss events linked to humiliation were the category of life events most likely to lead to major depression, thereby providing support for the proposed sadness–self-disgust (in the form of shame and humiliation) link proposed here. Finally, in order to explore the potential roles of guilt and shame, Massimo Tarsia and I carried out a study of a group of individuals presenting to a psychology clinic with problems with depression, anxiety, or both (Power and Tarsia, 2007). Among a number of procedures, they were asked to complete the Basic Emotions Scale (Power, 2006). In statistical analyses, we found that both the recent self-reported levels of guilt and the levels of shame (or self-disgust) were correlated with the severity of depression when included separately in the regression analyses, but only the level of shame remained predictive when they were included together.

That is, shame rather than guilt is more important, both statistically and conceptually, in relation to depression. Shame of course is a much more all-encompassing and aversive emotion than guilt, but the fact that DSM and ICD have missed its importance in depression and in other types of psychopathology adds to their already long list of limitations, as reviewed in Chapter 2.

Disgust Disorders

A summary of the basic, complex, and coupled emotions associated with disgust are shown in Table 6.7. The role of disgust is related initially to specific physical survival drives that include repulsion toward certain tastes and smells, which eventually develop into repulsion and rejection of certain foodstuffs and bodily products. Hence, as with anxiety, disgust initially has a protective function, but with more focus on food and bodily products. This physical function then develops with the appearance of the "self-conscious" emotions such as guilt and shame in which the actions of the self and even the self itself can become the focus of the emotion (e.g., Tangney, 1999). These self-disgust emotions can play a part in a wide range of psychopathology, as we have discussed in other sections and chapters, though the ones that we especially wish to highlight are the coupling with anxiety in certain phobias and obsessions and with sadness in depression.

We noted in the section on anxiety disorders that some types of phobias are more likely to be disgust-based or reflect disgust–anxiety coupling than they are simply anxiety-based. For example, in countries where there are no poisonous spiders, the reaction to the harmless spider in the bath is more of a disgust reaction than it is of an anxiety reaction, with the feeling that the spider has contaminated the bath making

Table 6.7: Drive–emotion–cognition (DEC) analysis of disgust disorders.

Drive	Emotion	Cognition
Survival drives –Physical –Social	(Basic) Disgust	Contamination Repulsion
Survival drives –Physical –Social	(Complex) Guilt Shame	Contamination Self-repulsion
Survival drives –Physical –Social	(Coupled) Sadness–disgust Anxiety–disgust	Self-repulsion Threat Contamination

it difficult for the person to use the bath without excessive cleaning even after the spider has been removed. Reactions to other creatures that can be dangerous, such as snakes, are likely to involve a mix of anxiety and disgust rather than just anxiety alone. It is clear also that the drop of blood pressure, bradycardia, and risk of fainting that accompany disgust reactions are present in blood–injury–injection phobias in contrast to anxiety-based phobias in which an increase in blood pressure and tachycardia make it *less* likely that the person will faint. It also seems likely that social phobia is likely to be characterized by a coupling of anxiety and shame, because of the fear of being shamed in a range of social situations (Beck and Emery, 1985).

We also noted in the section on anxiety disorders that although some types of OCD are more likely to be anxiety-based (e.g., those that involve checking), the contamination and washing-based types of OCD are more likely to be disgust-based. Evidence has now begun to accumulate in favor of a role for disgust in some types of OCD, following our proposal for such in an earlier book (Power and Dalgleish, 1997). Phillips et al. (2000) in a functional magnetic resonance imaging (fMRI) study of people with washer versus checker types of OCD found specific activation of the insula for washer-relevant disgust pictures (e.g., urinals, rubbish bags), but both washers and checkers showed elevated insula activation for general disgust pictures (e.g., wounds, cockroaches, decaying food) compared with controls. Studies that have already found association in non-clinical populations have also shown correlations in clinical populations between disgust sensitivity and obsessional symptoms, especially related to washing (Mancini et al., 2001). A fMRI study by Shapira et al. (2003) of eight OCD patients with contamination fears showed similar activation compared with healthy controls for threat (anxiety) pictures; they only differed from controls for disgust pictures and again showed increased activation of the insula. Taken together, the evidence is beginning to point to a useful distinction between disgust and fear in the etiology and maintenance of different types of OCD.

The role of self-disgust in depression captures an important aspect of the disorder that simply seeing depression as a disorder of sadness fails to recognize, as we argued in the section Sadness Disorders. Although both guilt and shame are self-focused complex emotions derived from disgust, the traditional DSM focus has been on guilt; however, in a statistical analysis of the emotions of guilt and shame in clinical depression we found that shame was the more important emotion in the prediction of the severity of depression (Power and Tarsia, 2007). There is now increasing evidence for the role of shame in depression (e.g., Gilbert, 2013).

Disgust is still a relatively under-researched emotion, especially in its putative role in a range of disorders stretching from phobias, to OCD, to depression, to eating disorders, to some types of PTSD. It forms the basis not only of basic reactions to food and bodily products but also provides the foundation for morality and the moral judgments that we make about ourselves and others (Rozin and Fallon, 1987). As such, the role of disgust and self-disgust in psychological disorders deserves increased consideration.

Happiness Disorders

Well we have saved the best until last, in good biblical tradition. As we have commented elsewhere, in societies where the pursuit of happiness has become such an overvalued commodity, the idea of happiness disorder can, at least superficially, appear somewhat strange (Power, in press). Perhaps it is because, in Western society, we are more tolerant of variations and extremes within the parameters, both cognitive and physiological, that define a particular individual's positive emotions, and are thus less likely to "label" the emotion as disordered in comparison with the cases of extreme variants of negative emotions such as anger, fear, or sadness. In other, non-Western, cultures happiness or joy are regarded are far less socially acceptable than in the West. For example, the Ifaluk, a small Micronesian culture, equate happiness with a tendency for the individual to disregard others and the needs of the social group (Lutz, 1988). For the Ifaluk, then, happiness is a negative emotion, whereas sadness is encouraged as a positive emotional state. Despite the paucity of discussion on abnormal happiness in the literature, we propose that extreme variations in the cognitive or physiological parameters that contribute to the emotion of happiness may be usefully conceptualized as types of "happiness disorder," with a summary across basic, complex, and coupled emotions derived from happiness presented in Table 6.8.

Table 6.8: Drive–emotion–cognition analysis of happiness disorders.

Drive	Emotion	Cognition
Attachment	(Basic)	Success
Domination	Happiness	Achievement
Survival		Connection
Attachment	(Complex)	Triumph
Domination	Pride	Connection
Survival	Love	Intimacy
Attachment	(Coupled)	Superiority
Domination	Happiness–anxiety	Grandiosity
Survival	Happiness–anger	Creativity
	Love–anxiety	Love-sick
	Love–sadness	

Perhaps the disorders that seem most clearly to be ones of happiness or positive mood are hypomania and mania. The central features are elevation of mood, hyperactivity, and grandiose ideas about the self (e.g., Jauhar and Cavanagh, 2013). Manic individuals often seem cheerful and optimistic when their mood is elevated and have an infectious gaiety. However, other individuals can be irritable rather than euphoric, and their emotions are extremely labile so that this irritability can easily translate into anger. There is often diurnal variation in the individual's mood, whether it be irritable or euphoric. However, this variation does not normally conform to the regular patterns of other depressive disorders. Even in patients who are elated, it is not unusual for their periods of elevated mood to be interrupted by brief episodes of depression, and in fact these "mixed state" presentations in mania, in which there may be a range of emotions present, seem to be much more typical than previously considered (Cassidy and Carroll, 2001). Manic individuals commonly experience expansive ideas. They believe that their thoughts and ideas are original, their opinions important, and their work of the most outstanding quality. Occasionally these expansive themes merge into grandiose delusions in which the individual believes he or she is a religious prophet or a famous person. Such grandiosity and expansiveness also manifest in extravagant behavior; manic individuals often spend more than they can afford, make reckless decisions, give up good jobs, or embark on schemes and ventures which have little chance of success. Such problems are compounded by impaired insight in most cases. Manic individuals will often see no reason why their grandiose plans should be reined in or their extravagant expenditure curtailed. Manic individuals rarely think of themselves as having an emotional problem or needing any kind of help while they are manic.

In mania and hypomania, it appears that the individual's dominant schematic models of self are highly self-serving, leading to the setting of unrealistic and optimistic goals. The achievement of these goals, or the belief that they have been achieved, is a source of joy and elation. There seems to be little or no access to the representations of the goals of others and, most notably, the shared goals of self and others—the social standards that are so important for setting limits on behavior. Allied with this is the manic person's tendency to switch from periods of extreme gaiety to periods of intense anger or depression. It seems that different configurations of self-related schematic models come to dominate and regulate the system, such that at one moment everything is all rosy and the next it is all black. The tendency for mania and hypomania to co-occur with depression provides a difficult challenge that no biological or psychological theory has effectively accounted for. One might speculate that, first, if the self becomes predominantly organized around issues of success versus failure, appraisals of goal attainment versus goal failure for a highly invested domain are very likely to occur at different points (e.g., Power et al., 2002), so the person may swing between the emotions of joy, sadness, and self-disgust accordingly.

Disorders of love provide another interesting area of challenge in our love-preoccupied society (see the enjoyable book by Frank Tallis (2004), *Love Sick: Love as a Mental Illness*). The idea that our "choice" of lover is also somehow a function of our attachment processes is clearly not a new one, and is a fundamental concept in psychodynamic psychology (e.g., Bowlby, 1988). For many people, this choice is likely to be a functional one. The potential lover often has qualities that would also make them a good partner in a loving relationship over the long term. However, for other individuals the people who rouse their passions are exactly the sort of people who their rational thoughts tell them should be avoided. Furthermore, as we mentioned in Chapter 5 on social drives, for the majority of individuals the choice of lover is partly a function of the likelihood that the chosen person will reciprocate their feelings. However, for others, there is often a pattern of falling in love with people when the chances of a reciprocated loving relationship are small or even non-existent. This problem is manifest, in its most extreme form, in the disorder of erotomania, or De Clerambault's syndrome, in which individuals fall in love with public figures or famous personages who they are unlikely even to meet (e.g., Franzini and Grossberg, 1995). A sobering example of this is the case of John Hinckley, mentioned in Chapter 2, who attempted to assassinate Ronald Reagan in 1981 as a last-ditch attempt to impress the actress Jodie Foster with whom he reported being desperately in love.

A final point that we want to make in this section on happiness disorders is to come back to a point that we raised in Chapter 4 on disorders of drives when we speculated that although it might seem reasonable to classify drug and alcohol disorders as drive-related or appetitive disorders, it might also be worthwhile considering if, instead, they could be a type of emotional disorder. A similar argument could also be applied to the gambling disorders. Of course, issues of physical and psychological dependence complicate discussions of drug and alcohol problems; nevertheless, many drug, alcohol, and gambling problems seem to have their basis in issues of emotion regulation, with attempts to induce positive emotion states and remove negative emotions providing key perpetuating factors for the disorders. The disorders can of course be multiply determined with drive-related (e.g., suppression of appetite, increasing wakefulness, increased sexual performance, etc.), emotion-related (induction of positive affect, removal of negative affect), and cognition-related (e.g., increased creativity, improved concentration) onset and maintenance factors, all of which could apply at different times, such as in the effects of smoking in nicotine dependence. Nevertheless, we now believe there could be considerable benefit from taking an emotion-focused approach to the understanding of such disorders.

Summary and Conclusions

In this chapter we have reviewed how the five basic emotions of anger, anxiety, sadness, disgust, and happiness form the basis of our emotional lives, in that elaborations, blends, and coupling of these five emotions provide the basis for emotional experience across individuals' lives and across all cultures. As we have shown, the experience of an emotion such as panic can be taken as evidence of a disorder by one person, whereas the "same" experience can be viewed simply as a somewhat unpleasant emotional state by another. The "emotion disorders" therefore highlight very clearly the important constructive aspect of the psychological disorders that we have emphasized throughout this book, namely, that the same experience can be construed as either normality or as madness depending on a variety of personal, familial, religious, and cultural belief systems. One of the main aims of the range of talking therapies that have been developed for working with the emotional disorders has been to help people reconstrue their anxiety-provoking "mad" experiences to come within the normal range of experience and thereby improve their regulation and management. Of course, as we will see in Chapter 7, one of the classic diagnostic arguments between psychiatry and psychology has been whether people with such anxiety disorders should simply be classified as the "worried well," whose experiences fall within the normal range, or "genuinely mad," that is people who suffer from severe delusions and hallucinations and for the past 100 years have been labeled as suffering from "schizophrenia" or something similar. We will return to this issue in Chapter 7 when we outline the various disorders that can be considered as primarily disorders of cognition.

7

DISORDERS OF COGNITION

The people who are crazy enough to think they can change the world are the ones who do

Apple, Inc.

Introduction

In this chapter we will examine what can be labeled primarily as disorders of cognition, though like all the disorders considered throughout this book each includes aspects of drives and emotions to a lesser or greater extent, and these will also be examined. The approach that will be taken for understanding cognition is to break it down into a set of cognitive mechanisms or processes in the standard manner used by textbooks on cognitive science, that is, perception and attention, thinking and reasoning, memory, language, and motor skills. Each of these systems is potentially dissociable from the other systems in that there may be dedicated functional processors for each. Of course, further dissociations are apparent even within these broader systems, such as the division of memory into different subsystems of short-term memory and long-term memory, different sensory-based perceptual systems, and so on (e.g., Eysenck and Keane, 2010). Such use of a cognitive domains or cognitive systems approach has also been considered within DSM-5, in that a similar set of cognitive domains to those considered here are suggested to cut across the various neurocognitive disorders, with assessment of neurocognitive functioning being recommended in specific cognitive domains.

One of the issues that occurs for each of the cognitive disorders is the question of "belief about" dysfunction versus "actual" dysfunction, an issue that has been raised in previous chapters but is of equal importance for cognitive disorders. For example, many older adults who present themselves for assessment in memory clinics believe that they may be suffering from some form of memory impairment because they may be aware of problems with memory retrieval for names, faces, general knowledge, and so on. Although difficulties with memory retrieval occur at all ages and for a variety of reasons other than organic memory impairment, a substantial number of older adults can become worried that they may be suffering from early signs of dementia even though their memory performance is normative for their age (e.g., Hejl et al., 2002). Some colleagues in some professions might wish to label such individuals as the "worried well" rather than "genuinely mad." However, such a view is mistaken and overly simplistic in its approach to psychological disorders in that many disorders consist of a mix of belief and experience, the interaction of which can either exacerbate the problem or, in contrast, lead to the "problem" being managed in an optimal way, as summarized in the two-by-two table in Table 7.1.

The modern battle, sometimes labeled as psychiatry versus antipsychiatry, is the one fought over the concept of schizophrenia and whether or not it is a genuine disorder, a social construct, or a means of political control (e.g., Boyle, 2002). Because of its recent and continuing importance, we will begin this chapter on cognitive disorders with a detailed consideration of the concept of schizophrenia. However, before we even start the discussion we have to begin by saying that the concept of schizophrenia as identified in the DSM and ICD systems cannot exist! The problem, as we will show in detail, is that from a cognitive systems point of view the diagnostic approaches to "schizophrenia" mistakenly conflate perceptual/attentional systems with thinking/reasoning systems, when, as we have already noted, these are dissociable. In plainer English, the defining symptoms for schizophrenia can either be perceptual/attentional, with auditory hallucinations being the most common, or thinking/reasoning based, with delusions and elaborated delusional systems being the most common. However, our cognitive science-based separation of perceptual/attentional systems as distinct from thinking/reasoning systems provides very different cognitive mechanisms for hallucinations versus delusions and would not begin by defining a single disorder such as "schizophrenia" that can be based on either one or the other. Hallucinations can and do occur without delusions, just as delusions can and do occur without hallucinations. While the two systems can overlap, in that for example people may come to have unusual beliefs about their hallucinations, correlation does not imply cause and therefore the traditional concept of schizophrenia must be dismantled even before we have come to review it in detail.

Table 7.1: Possible outcomes for belief and experience in disorders.

	Experience absent	Experience present
Belief—positive	Healthy	Managed
Belief—negative	Vulnerable	Disordered

Table 7.2: Drive–emotion–cognition summary of cognitive systems.

Drive	Emotion	Cognition
Memory system	Anxiety (etc.)	Memory problems
Perception/attention system		Perception/attention problems
Thinking/reasoning system		Thinking/reasoning problems
Motor system		Motor problems
Language system		Language problems

Table 7.2 presents a summary of the categories that we will use in this chapter for disorders of cognition together with typical associated drive- and emotion-related problems. These categories cover perception/attention, thinking/reasoning, memory, language, and motor skills and we will consider examples of both functional and organic impairment, though we will concentrate primarily on the functional disorders because they are the focus of this book. The organic disorders will be noted in passing, in particular where they have contributed to an increase in understanding of the cognitive systems. We will begin with the impairments in perception and attention and some of the considerable controversies to which they have led.

Disorders of Perception/Attention

In this section we will launch straight into the problematic diagnostic category of "schizophrenia." As discussed in Chapters 1 and 2, the term was introduced by the Swiss psychiatrist Eugen Bleuler in 1911. It replaced Emil Kraepelin's "dementia praecox" and has subsequently been used in preference to Kraepelin's term in order to avoid the implication that schizophrenia is a dementia-like disease with progressive deterioration. Instead, "schizophrenia" referred to a split in thinking in which, in associative psychology terms, normal associations between ideas and between ideas and emotions are broken (note that this usage does not imply the "split personality" that has crept into the depictions by Hollywood and the media). Bleuler's term therefore did not imply any inevitable deterioration in a disease process, with the implication in fact that recovery should be possible for at least some sufferers.

The most recent revision of the category of "schizophrenia" as presented in DSM-5 is shown in Table 7.3. As noted above, the categories of delusions, hallucinations, disorganized speech, disorganized or catatonic behavior, and negative symptoms derive from different and dissociable cognitive systems. To focus on the categories of delusions and hallucinations: a cognitive systems analysis shows that one can have hallucinations without delusions, and delusions without hallucinations. Of course,

Table 7.3: Main symptoms of schizophrenia from DSM-5.

	Symptoms—at least two from criterion A
A1	Delusions
A2	Hallucinations
A3	Disorganized speech
A4	Disorganized or catatonic behavior
A5	Negative symptoms (reduced emotional expression, avolition)
B	Reduced psychosocial functioning
C	Signs of disturbance for at least 6 months

in order to explain their hallucinations some people may develop abnormal beliefs that appear to be delusional; but these beliefs are developed in response to extreme experiences such as auditory hallucinations. A statement of the belief "I hear the voice of God" could be considered to be delusional, but in theory it should be possible to challenge such a belief and offer an alternative explanation for the hallucination (e.g., Garety and Hemsley, 1994). Equally, it is possible for an individual to develop an elaborate delusional system without any hallucinations, yet still be given the label "schizophrenia" under the DSM-5 diagnostic criteria.

Evidence for this proposed splitting of schizophrenia into at least two different disorders comes from a number of studies. Although, as noted by Mellers et al. (1996), many previous factor analytic studies of the symptoms of schizophrenia found support for Peter Liddle's (1987) three factors, for one of which delusions and hallucinations load together, these authors argued that such findings arise from studies of longer-term *chronic* schizophrenia. In their study Mellers and colleagues examined symptom presentation on the Present State Examination of 114 patients with *acute* schizophrenia who had just been admitted to hospital and who met the DSM-III-R criteria for schizophrenia. In this acute population they found that four factors fitted the data better, with delusions and hallucinations forming separate factors. Gunduz-Bruce et al. (2005) examined longitudinal time to response data for up to 5 years' follow up in 118 participants who met the criteria for a first episode of schizophrenia, but in which they examined time to response for delusions and hallucinations separately. The authors found that time to response for delusions was significantly longer than time to response for hallucinations. Furthermore, whereas time to the start of treatment was predictive of time to response for delusions, in which a longer duration of non-treatment predicted a longer time to response, no such relationship was found for hallucinations. There is also evidence that pathways into the experience of hallucinations in adulthood may be different from those that lead to delusions; thus, Read et al. (2003) found that childhood sexual abuse was associated with the presence of hallucinations in adulthood, but only when combined with adult abuse was it also associated with delusions. Perhaps one of the mechanisms associated with the experience of childhood sexual abuse is the increase in use of dissociation, which may then later lead to an increased risk of hallucinatory experience in that some experiences come to be experienced as "not-self" and therefore split off from the self as if they were externally generated (Power and Dalgleish, 2008).

The suggestion, therefore, is that *some* people who go on to develop symptoms that fit the DSM category of "schizophrenia" develop unusual beliefs about their hallucinatory experiences whereas others do not. Evidence for such a process comes, for example, from a study by Smeets et al. (2010) which involved a 10-year follow-up study of a representative sample of 2524 adolescents and young adults in Munich. The authors identified four different groups of participants: (1) those without delusions or hallucinations, (2) those with isolated hallucinations, (3) those with isolated delusions, and (4) those with both delusions and hallucinations. The group with both delusions and hallucinations had the worst outcome and the greatest persistence of psychotic-like symptoms over the time course of the study. Furthermore, Smeets and colleagues found that the content of the delusions was related to the type of hallucinations but not vice versa, which suggests a mechanism whereby the development of delusional explanations in response to hallucinatory experiences is likely to have the worst outcome in terms of persistence of symptoms and greater use of health services.

The argument therefore is that if the disorders of cognition are to be based on and derived from the key cognitive systems, the dismantling of "schizophrenia" should lead to at least two, and possibly more, cognitive system disorders:

1. Hallucinations (hallucinatory disorder)—a perceptual/attentional disorder that typically includes auditory hallucinations, but that can also range across other sensory systems including visual, tactile, and olfactory systems. These hallucinatory disorders should be seen on a continuum, because such experiences in the absence of sensory input can occur under a wide range of normal conditions including falling asleep (hypnagogic hallucinations), waking from sleep (hypnopompic hallucinations), and of course in the hallucinations

that occur in dreams themselves. In fact there are now a number of interesting cognitive theories that consider hallucinations to reflect the operation of a top-down cognitive modeling system that under certain conditions can either operate in the absence of sensory input as in the case of dreams (see, e.g., Domhoff, 2003), or sometimes offer distortions of minimal sensory input as in Daniel Collerton's (e.g., Collerton and Taylor, 2013) account of the occurrence of visual hallucinations in a wide variety of conditions. Now one of the questions that arises with hallucinations is whether or not they are equivalent or need further specification along the lines of "schizophrenia-type hallucinations," "grief-type hallucinations," "dream-type hallucinations," and so on (Dave Hemsley, personal communication). That is, and in contrast to Richard Bentall's (e.g., Bentall, 2009) approach, it may be insufficient to lump together all hallucinations irrespective of a further specification of their possible etiology because they may differ in important ways from each other. However, a further possibility is that the DEC analysis of different types of hallucinations may be sufficient to provide differentiation between types of hallucinations; thus, the type of hallucination, the beliefs about the hallucination, the emotions linked to the hallucination, and the possible drive system associated with the hallucination should provide sufficient detail to answer Dave Hemsley's criticism of Richard Bentall's approach. Further theoretical and empirical study of hallucinations will be necessary in order to resolve this issue, but for now the psychosis-related hallucinations which are typically auditory in nature can be referred to as hallucinatory disorder. In the tradition of Kraepelin and Bleuler one could at this point set out to invent a new Greek- or Latin-derived name for such hallucinatory disorders, but we will leave such neologistic pursuits for others (those who remember sufficient Greek and Latin from their schooldays) to have fun with.

2. Delusions (delusional disorder)—the DSM already includes a separate category of "delusional disorder," which in DSM-IV emphasized that the delusions should be "non-bizarre" in order to distinguish them from delusions in schizophrenia, though this "non-bizarre" requirement has been dropped in DSM-5, which now includes "bizarre" as one of the possible specifiers of the disorder. The stand-alone delusions in DSM delusional disorder are further specified as:

   i. Erotomanic—in which the person believes that another person, typically someone of high status, is in love with them, a disorder that we previously considered as a love-related disorder sometimes referred to as De Clerambault's syndrome (see Chapter 6).

   ii. Grandiose—in which people believe that they may have a great talent or that they are a very important person. Such delusions are typically associated with bipolar disorder and can be most apparent in the manic phase (see Chapter 6).

   iii. Jealous—in which the person believes that his or her spouse is unfaithful despite all the evidence being to the contrary. Again we would see this as an emotional disorder rather than primarily a cognitive disorder.

   iv. Persecutory—when the person believes that he or she is being conspired against in some extreme way, despite evidence to the contrary.

   v. Somatic—for example, the belief that the body emits a foul smell, or is misshapen or infected in some way.

One observation about the majority of these delusional subtypes is that they all have a strong emotional content (cf. Garety et al., 2001), but they range across the basic emotions from anxiety to anger to happiness and they also have strong drive-related components. The DEC analyses of many of these delusions seem very appropriate. However, we would go one step further and argue that there is a logical inconsistency within the DSM system in that while the delusional disorder has been separated out from schizophrenia, the hallucinatory disorder has not. The DSM experts seem to have taken only the first step toward dismantling the "schizophrenia" portmanteau construct, but for DSM-6 they should take the next essential step and divide it into at least two separate disorders, based on specified cognitive systems.

Disorders of Thinking/Reasoning

The proposed division of "schizophrenia" into an attention/perception disorder and a thinking/reasoning disorder has already provided a starting point for our discussion of possible disorders of thinking and reasoning, in that delusional beliefs provide input to thinking and reasoning from which unusual or bizarre conclusions may be drawn by the individual, for example in order to resist challenges to those extreme beliefs. Of course, one of the problems with elaborated delusional systems is, to put it crudely: if one person believes it then it is labeled as madness, but if a group of people believe it then it can become a cult or a religion. As an example, let us consider the Heaven's Gate movement that I have discussed previously (Power, 2012). Marshall Applewhite (1931–97) founded the Heaven's Gate movement with his nurse, Bonnie Nettles (1928–85), following a heart attack and a near-death experience (NDE) in the 1970s. Applewhite believed that he and Nettles were extraterrestrial beings from another world that represented "the evolutionary level above human" and that they had been planted on the garden of Earth to help other humans mature to this higher evolutionary level. In order to achieve this higher level, followers had to relinquish their animal selves, including their sexuality, such that many of the men in the movement, including Applewhite, castrated themselves. In March 1997, Applewhite claimed that the appearance of the Hale–Bopp comet was the arrival of the spaceship to collect them, following which the apocalyptic end of the Earth would occur. On March 26, 1997 police found the bodies of Applewhite and 38 followers on a ranch near San Diego; they had all committed suicide and were all wearing armbands saying "Heaven's Gate away team."

The problem with examples such as the Heaven's Gate movement, and indeed the extraordinary beliefs that can be seen in all religious movements, is that as a species we have developed some extraordinary and diverse beliefs about the universe around us and our potential role within it (Power, 2012). These belief systems include most of the possible psychosis-related phenomena, and many other phenomena besides. For example, the NDE that was crucial in Marshall Applewhite's development of the Heaven's Gate movement provides the central focus for Gregory Shushan in his book *Conceptions of the Afterlife in Early Civilizations* (Shushan, 2009) in which he argues that there is a considerable uniformity among largely unconnected ancient cultures regarding belief in life after death and that the core elements of these religious beliefs are largely similar to those of NDEs. In his book, Shushan examines conceptions of the afterlife in ancient Egypt, Mesopotamia, China (before the arrival of Buddhism), India (also before the arrival of Buddhism), and pre-Columbian Mesoamerica. Shushan compares the afterlife accounts in each of these five civilizations and concludes that the differences between the afterlife experiences in ancient texts and the NDE accounts are predominately at the symbolic, culture-specific level but that, "the NDE itself appears to be a collection of subjectively experienced universal phenomena." Shushan summarizes a number of key elements of NDEs that form the basis for afterlife conceptions in these early civilizations that include:

an out-of-body experience
corpse encounters, for example with dead relatives (ancestors)
the experience of passing through darkness or a tunnel
passing into the presence of intense light
an experience of union (oneness) and enlightenment
the feeling of being in another realm or at the point of origin.

Shushan argues very persuasively that NDEs were clearly part of the experience of these ancient cultures and that they provided key evidence for the nature of the afterlife in an otherwise diverse set of religious beliefs and practices. For example, he argues that in contrast to conceptions of the afterlife, these same ancient cultures have extremely diverse accounts of creation or creation myths ("cosmogonies") because there is no shared experiential basis from which to develop a culture's creation myths. The key point for our consideration of possible psychological disorders is that experiences that could be labeled as psychotic (thought removal, soul removal, thought insertion, soul insertion, demonic possession, in addition to a range of auditory and visual hallucinations that provide "evidence" for the existence of supernatural beings) have often formed the pillars of religious and other related belief systems and would be endorsed in one form or another by a very large proportion of the world's cultures.

A third aspect of the DSM-5 criteria for schizophrenia shown in Table 7.3 is that of the category "thought disorder," but in DSM-5 this has been articulated as disorganized speech and disorganized or catatonic behavior. Thought disorder is yet another omnibus category that could arise from non-optimal processing in at least one cognitive mechanism, though it is likely to represent multiple non-optimal processes interacting with each other. For example, work on executive functioning from at least Norman and Shallice (1980) onwards has highlighted the crucial role that an executive mechanism plays in a range of planning, control, timing, inhibition, updating, shifting, and retrieval functions, such that these functions appear to run smoothly and coherently when the system is operating optimally. However, there are a range of factors that can impact on executive functioning and the capacity of working memory, including stress, emotion, multitasking demands, illness, fatigue, and degeneration. In fact Baddeley (1996) suggested that there could be a *dysexecutive syndrome* in which damage to the frontal lobes can lead to a variety of problems with planning, inhibition, monitoring, and overall organization of behavior. A number of such deficits that have been identified in people diagnosed with schizophrenia (e.g., Frommann et al., 2011) have led some people to argue that in addition to separate dimensions or factors of hallucinations and delusions, there is a third separate factor of *thought disorder* that can be identified from factor analyses of the symptoms of schizophrenia and that is also present in factor analyses of more general symptomatology across a wide range of disorders (e.g., Kotov et al., 2011). The fact that *thought disorder* emerges in a wide range of psychopathologies points to its origins in the impact on high-level cognitive processes of a range of drive-, emotion-, and cognition-related psychopathologies that is not therefore unique to the diagnosis of schizophrenia. Nevertheless, it seems likely that the extent of the thought disorder is a reflection of the severity of the other psychopathology that leads to an increasing impact on executive and other cognitive functions.

Therefore the approach that must be taken to a discussion of potential disorders of thinking/reasoning is that they must lie on one or more continua, given that most people share at least some objectively bizarre beliefs from which various objectively bizarre conclusions can be reasonably drawn because they are based on faith rather than on evidence (Power, 2012). Delusional disorders are not therefore qualitatively distinct, but lie on a continuum with other belief systems, a proportion of which may also cause distress to the holder of the beliefs or may put at risk either the holder of the beliefs or people around them. For example, although we considered anorexia in Chapter 4 as a drive disorder and OCD in Chapter 6 as an emotional disorder, both of these can present with beliefs that verge on the extreme and can sometimes be considered "delusional" and are highly resistant to any form of intervention or challenge. In DSM-5 one of the specifiers for OCD is the degree of insight the person has into his or her beliefs: (1) good or fair insight, (2) poor insight, or (3) absent insight/delusional beliefs. Although divided into three categories, the specifier represents a dimensional evaluation of how much insight the OCD sufferer has into the obsessions and compulsions and the beliefs surrounding their activity, though relatively few people with OCD fall into the absent insight group compared with those with body dysmorphic disorder, for example (Phillips et al., 2012). Examples of the types of dysfunctional beliefs that OCD sufferers may have include excessive responsibility, overestimation of threat, perfectionism, intolerance of uncertainty, and excessive need for control of thoughts. However, many of these types of thoughts, although more prevalent in OCD than in healthy controls, are not unique to OCD but can be elevated in other anxiety disorders and in depression. Thus, when an OCD group was compared with an anxiety control group and the level of depression was controlled for Tolin et al. (2006) found that only beliefs about the need to control one's thoughts were higher in the OCD group.

The actual thoughts that OCD sufferers have can be quite unique in any particular case; for example, one man I worked with had stopped using his motorbike because while he was riding it he constantly thought that there was a trail of dead bodies behind him and he spent much of his time going back to check on whether or not this was true. He had little or no insight into the veracity of his thoughts, which is why he had stopped motorcycling altogether.

A similar issue about extreme and dysfunctional beliefs can also be found in anorexia, an overlap that has led some to suggest that there could be a relationship between the two disorders of anorexia and OCD. The issue of insight into beliefs and the degree of delusionality of beliefs arises again. Konstantakopoulos et al. (2013) assessed the degree of delusionality of the body beliefs in a group of 39 people with anorexia and 33 with bulimia. Whereas 28.8% of the anorexia group were rated as having delusional body beliefs, none of the bulimia group was given such a rating. Of course, as with OCD the dysfunctional beliefs that can be found in anorexia range widely from body-related beliefs, to beliefs about food, control, and avoidance of thoughts and emotions, and interpersonal relations (Fox and Power, 2009; Treasure and Schmidt, 2013).

The overall message from this section on disorders of thinking and reasoning is that a wide variety of psychological disorders can include some form of thought disorder, in that an optimally functioning cognitive system can be disrupted by a wide range of factors. However, even apparently delusional beliefs that would in the past have only been considered in relation to psychosis can now be found in other non-psychotic disorders, including examples in OCD and anorexia. The point is that belief systems need to be considered on dimensions of rigidity and fixedness, otherwise many socially shared belief systems would meet the criteria for delusionality. Such a change in views about belief systems is reflected in the increasing emphasis within recent diagnostic systems such as DSM-5 on degree of insight ratings, that range from complete to absent or delusional, for beliefs that impact on a range of disorders, not just the schizophreniform ones.

Disorders of Memory

Although one might at first only think of memory disorders that are based on organic impairment, for example the dementias, there are also a number of functional disorders of memory that must also be considered. Indeed, the whole question of *false memories* and the return of *repressed memories* has been an area of great controversy for a number of decades (e.g., Davies and Dalgleish, 2001).

Perhaps one of the more intriguing aspects of the whole literature on false memory has to be the reports of alien abduction. If these increasing numbers of claims are to be believed, then it is estimated that several thousand Americans are *each day* taken aboard fleets of spaceships hovering somewhere over the Mid-West of the USA where lengthy medical examinations are carried out by groups of intergalactic physicians. The abducted individuals are then returned to their humdrum lives and only manage to recall these abduction episodes using memory recovery techniques such as hypnosis. In their studies of these phenomena, Newman and Baumeister (1998) observed that about 80% of abductions occur in the USA, with virtually none being reported in Asia and Africa. Newman and Baumeister have also noted an increasing trend toward reported sexual interference from the alien abductors. If we can assume that there is no such fleet of extraterrestrial, NASA, or Hollywood spacecraft, these reports of alien abduction are surely proof that individuals can recover "memories" of events that have never occurred. They are proof that suggestible individuals, when placed under the influence of credible experts such as therapists, are vulnerable to the recovery of false memories. The question concerning false memory therefore becomes not *whether* but *how* and *when*.

The other side of the argument about false memory is whether or not a memory can be forgotten for a long period of time and then subsequently recovered. We need to ask whether or not *traumatic* events (i.e., events that would be judged by most as difficult if not impossible to forget because of their nature) can in fact be forgotten. In addition, do special intrapsychic mechanisms such as "repression" need to be mooted to explain such forgetting or can such forgetting can be accounted for by the characteristics of remembering and forgetting, about which everyone would agree. The preliminary framework for examining the issues around recovered memories is presented in Table 7.4 and is taken from Power (2001).

Table 7.4 is adapted from one in which we previously considered some of the conditions under which an individual's accuracy in judgment and reasoning tasks varies according to the truth value of the information (i.e., true or false), the valence of the information (i.e., positive or negative), and the mood state of the individual (e.g., normal or depressed) (Power and Dalgleish, 2008). On reasoning and judgment tasks there is evidence that depressed individuals may be more accurate in accepting true negatives and rejecting false positives, whereas normal non-depressed individuals may be more accurate at rejecting false negatives and accepting true positives. The application of this framework to recovered memory as shown in Table 7.4 suggests that each of the equivalent four categories need to be considered, that is, true remembered, true recovered, false remembered, and false recovered. By summarizing information about each of these four categories we can obtain useful illustrations of the operation of memory under different conditions.

1. *True remembered memories.* This is the major category that most people associate with memory. Memory is widely assumed to be an accurate and veridical process—a long-standing tradition that includes Freud among its proponents (e.g., Freud, 1900). Perhaps Freud's influence may be one reason why Loftus

Table 7.4: The status of memories.

	Remembered	Recovered
True	True memory	Repressed
False	Memory error	False memory

and Loftus (1980) obtained the astonishing finding that over 80% of therapists when surveyed stated that they believed all memories to be permanently recorded in the brain. However, the tradition in memory research that stems from the work of Bartlett (1932) presents a contrasting view of the process of memory. Bartlett studied memory for complex prose passages such as the famous "War of the Ghosts" story over extended periods of time, even to the extent of reputedly jumping off his bicycle in the middle of Cambridge years after the initial study and asking former participants to recall the text. Memory research in this tradition has demonstrated that memory can be surprisingly accurate over long periods of time, but in addition the process of retrieval is often a *reconstructive process* rather than simple retrieval (e.g., Neisser, 1976).

2. *True recovered memories.* The category that we have labeled "true recovered memories" refers to memories that although present in some form or other may remain inaccessible for long periods of time. This category is of course one of the most controversial of the four and is one about which (some) clinicians and experimentalists have been sharply divided (see, e.g., Davies and Dalgleish, 2001). The controversial version of the category of true recovered memories refers of course to the possibility of *active inhibitory* processes in memory. The best-known claims draw on Freud's (e.g., Freud, 1915) proposals for repression and infantile amnesia, but other dramatic examples relate to Janet's (e.g., Janet, 1889) accounts of *dissociative* rather than repressed states, seen for example in psychogenic amnesia and fugue states (see Chapter 8 of Kopelman and Morton, 2001). The reactions to Freud's ideas on repressed memories have included extreme responses such as Holmes' (1990) outright rejection of the possibility on the grounds that repression has never been demonstrated in the laboratory. Fortunately, for ethical reasons, there are limits to what can be done to participants in experiments in psychology laboratories and, just as in the case of neurological disorders, brain injury, etc., it is necessary to draw on single case studies that reflect "experiments of nature." More recent longitudinal studies of children who have experienced childhood sexual abuse and adult survivors of such abuse (e.g., Widom, 1997; Williams, 1995) have provided support for the possibility of repressed memories of sexual abuse. For example, Williams (1995) reported that in a group of children whose abuse had been corroborated a substantial proportion did not report the abuse when followed up many years later. In addition, there have now been demonstrations that a proportion of individuals possess a so-called repressive coping style (operationally defined as high scores on social desirability and low self-reported levels of anxiety; see, e.g., Weinberger et al., 1979). These individuals have been shown to have poor

recall of early negative memories (Myers and Brewin, 1994) together with poor recall of negative items on the Directed Forgetting Task (Myers et al., 1998). In summary, therefore, there are a number of potential mechanisms by which memories may apparently be forgotten over long periods of time, mechanisms that operate through active inhibitory processes. The mechanisms involved in directed forgetting, repression, dissociation, and mood-state-dependent effects demonstrate, both in the clinic and in the laboratory, that such active inhibitory processes occur. However, they do not guarantee that any such memory that has been forgotten and then remembered is necessarily true, as will be shown in the next two categories.

3. *False remembered memories.* One of the early examples of this category is probably represented in Freud's (1899) proposal for the existence of "screen memories." Freud argued that these memories were invariably wrong, at least if not in their entirety in some of the detail. He proposed that their function was literally to screen the individual against some earlier repressed memory to which the screen memory was linked in a meaningful way. One of the interesting pieces of evidence that Freud adduced in support of this proposal was the observation that many childhood memories occur as if one were observing oneself, but such self-perception is impossible, so therefore the memory must be false in at least some respects.

A considerable body of work has stemmed from Elizabeth Loftus' (e.g., Loftus and Zanni, 1975) work demonstrating that post-event questioning about incidents can lead the individual to incorporate information from the question into the memory of the incident. For example, a question such as "What color was the car that was parked on the left?" presupposes that there was a car parked on the left; in a range of eyewitness testimony studies subjects have been found to be prone to the incorporation of such information into their memories for the events. A second relevant area of laboratory research involves the study of "memory illusions." In a similar fashion to the demonstration of perceptual illusions, researchers such as Roediger and McDermott (1995) have found that with a word list containing associates of the word "sleep," subjects will report with considerable confidence that the word "sleep" appeared in the list even though it was never presented. Similar effects can be found with more complex prose (e.g., Brewer, 1974). Given that there is evidence that imagined events can be subsequently recalled as if they had occurred (see Loftus, 1998, for a summary), there must also now be scope for exploring the impact of the increased use of these media on the occurrence of false memories. Interestingly, the work on imaginary memories suggests that individuals who score high on measures of dissociative experiences are more likely to remember previously imagined events as if they were real ones (see Loftus, 1998).

4. *False recovered memories.* The most controversial category of all in recent years has been that of false recovered memories, that is, memories that are believed to be true by the individual, that are recalled as having been actively inhibited over some period of time, but which are eventually shown to be false (e.g., Gudjonsson, 2001). The controversy surrounding this category has involved the claims and counter-claims surrounding the issues of child sexual abuse and the possibility that certain techniques, such as the memory recovery techniques used in some types of therapies, may lead to "memory implantation." These controversies have focused around some of the high-profile legal cases, particularly in the USA, and the formation of false memory societies such as the British one that was surveyed by Gudjonsson. The results from Gudjonsson's survey of the British False Memory Society characterize some of the key issues. First, many of the recovered memories involve alleged sexual abuse that occurred before the age of 5 years and in some cases as young as in the first year of life. Secondly, the majority of these memories were claimed to have been forgotten and only later recovered. Thirdly, the majority of the recovered memories were recovered during therapy. The question then becomes: is it possible that a false memory can either be actively inhibited or experienced as such, then subsequently "recovered" by the individual? Several of the areas of research already reviewed have implications for the possibility of recovery of false memories. These areas include literature on reality monitoring, eyewitness testimony, directed forgetting, and memory illusions, all of which are relevant to the possibility of production of false memories. The literature on memory illusion, reality monitoring, and eyewitness testimony now shows some of the conditions under which partial or complete false memories can be produced, including demonstrations of the implantation of memories that participants believe are recovered childhood memories. For example, Loftus and her colleagues (e.g., Loftus and Pickrell, 1995; Loftus, 1998) have shown how false memories can be implanted in some individuals for imagined childhood events such as being "lost in a shopping mall" or "getting a finger caught in a mousetrap." These studies show that even under laboratory conditions it is possible to create false memories and a belief that they have been recovered after a long period of time.

A further area that is worth mentioning is that of *déjà vu* and other related experiences (e.g., *déjà entendu*, *déjà raconte*, and so on). These experiences provide interesting examples of what will be classified here as recovered false memories. The reason for this classification is that the *déjà vu* experience, as Ross (1991) proposed "is not a valid memory at all but only a misplaced emotional experience posing as a memory" [p. 198]. That is, the individual believes that there is a memory triggered by the current situation, a false memory that is accompanied by a feeling of strangeness similar to that of the re-experiencing of a recovered memory. Such experiences are rarely researched these days except as symptoms of organic pathology, but they also reveal aspects of the working of memory.

The final piece in the jigsaw of the current false memory controversy concerns the role of a powerful and significant other, such as a therapist, in the production of "recovered" false memories. This effect, in parallel to the "directed forgetting" effect mentioned earlier, might appropriately be labeled "directed remembering." For example, in their careful analyses of cases of recovered memories, Shobe and Schooler (2001) have shown that the false memories are typically "planted" at one or more early points in therapy and then subsequently "recovered" at later points. Although this usually occurs in individual therapy work with therapists using memory recovery procedures such as hypnosis, they have found that it can also occur in group therapy sessions, through reading material on multiple personality disorder (dissociative identity disorder in DSM-5 parlance), through the use of medication regimes, and so on. Shobe and Schooler suggest from their case analyses that a period of 2–12 months is needed from the initial suggestion to the eventual "recall" of the false memories in therapy. Such studies demonstrate dramatically the plasticity of memory and its reconstructive nature; they demonstrate too that it is often the most vulnerable individuals who are prone to the implantation of such false memories when in a dependent relationship. Nevertheless, the laboratory studies show that there are conditions under which we can all believe in what are actually false memories.

In summary, therefore, just as with cognitive systems for attention, perception, thinking, and reasoning, our mnemonic systems are vulnerable to a number of problems that point to and are a consequence of the very nature of the operation of those systems themselves. In particular, the *reconstructive* nature of mnemonic systems makes them vulnerable to false memory recall, and to repression or loss of memory, depending on a variety of individual and other factors. Again it is clear that functional problems with memory must be placed on a continuum. In addition the diagnostic systems do not usually consider stand-alone functional memory disorders, despite the coining of the term *false memory syndrome* by Peter Freyd, a mathematician who was accused of abuse by his daughter and who then founded the False Memory Syndrome

Foundation in 1992. Nevertheless, if the diagnostic systems are to be consistent with their approach of labeling the extreme point on a continuum as a disorder, then perhaps they ought to consider what such an extreme functional memory disorder would consist of. Instead, systems such as DSM-5 focus on the *neurocognitive disorders*, many of which can impact on the mnemonic systems and which therefore will be briefly considered next.

Neurocognitive Disorders and Memory

There are a wide range of neurocognitive disorders that can impact on memory, including traumatic brain injury, Alzheimer's disease, Parkinson's disease, Huntington's disease, and other types of dementias. Perhaps one of the most famous and widely studied of all individuals in the history of psychology was the unfortunate HM [Henry Molaison] who died in 2008 at the age of 82. He had a cycling accident at the age of 7 that is thought to have resulted in the epilepsy from which he subsequently suffered. In 1953, in an attempt to control the seizures, the neurosurgeon William Scoville carried out a bitemporal medial section that, among other things, removed the hippocampal areas in both lobes. Years of research then showed that HM was unable to form new long-term memories from short-term memory, but was able to recall long-term memories that had been laid down before the surgery. Additional work showed that he could learn new motor skills and that these could be retained for up to at least a year (Corkin, 1968). Cases such as that of HM have therefore pointed to the complexity of the memory systems and how they relate to each other, factors that need to be taken into account in the assessment of learning and memory in suspected cases of neurocognitive impairment.

One of the early clues to a range of neurocognitive disorders such as Alzheimer's disease is the presence of mild cognitive impairment (MCI) in which typically there are early signs of problems with memory and learning. Initial screening and assessment of people with suspected MCI can therefore be used to identify those who are at increased risk of going on to develop neurocognitive disorders (e.g., Petersen, 2004). Previous literature suggests that patients with MCI are less impaired in representing single feature information but show impairment in binding complex events where two or more features need to be combined (Swainson et al., 2001). Hence, it is likely that people with MCI in the early stages of Alzheimer's disease will perform more poorly on tasks combining emotional information from bimodal channels (faces and voices) but not necessarily show deficits in a single modality (only faces or only voices) (Hunter, 2011). Understanding to what extent problems in combining multisensory information might influence social interaction in people with cognitive impairment is the first step in designing successful interventions to help patients and their families with social functioning. It is also possible that multisensory integration of emotional information is one of the underlying deficits in patients who report changes in their social and emotional processing. For instance, studies investigating particular types of dementia have suggested that patients are impaired in their ability to understand the mental states of others and to identify emotions (McDonald and Flanagan, 2004). Such problems are consistent with more general executive functioning deficits of which mnemonic retrieval and new learning are important aspects.

Disorders of Language

As with memory, there tends to be a greater focus on the disorders of language that are consequent on neurocognitive disorders, whether of a developmental nature or acquired later in life. Nevertheless, a variety of psychological problems can have an impact on speech and language functioning and therefore require a brief mention. These disorders can present as somatic symptom disorders, or more specifically in DSM-5 as conversion disorder (see the discussion in Chapter 4), in which typically temporary problems occur with speech or language, such as in cases of aphonia, dysphonia, dysarthria, and stuttering, though onset of such disorders in adulthood can also be indicative of neurological insults and other medical conditions. Sinkiewicz et al. (2013) studied a group of 41 women with functional aphonia and found them to have significantly higher levels of anxiety and depression than control reference groups. In their review of "hysterical mutism," Schuster et al. (2011) found a higher prevalence in women, with a typical onset at the age of 30–40 following experience of a stressful event but with recovery occurring within about 3 months. What little is known about the language conversion disorders therefore points to the importance of stress and other emotion-related factors in their onset.

There are a number of learning disorders that are specifically neurodevelopmental, of which dyslexia is perhaps the most well known and widely researched. Dyslexia is a condition that becomes evident during the early school years and involves problems with fluency and comprehension during reading, though dyslexias can be acquired later in life following brain damage. A study by Whitehouse and Bishop (2009) examined dyslexia and anxiety in over 900 monozygotic and 900 dizygotic twin pairs. They found that although dyslexia and anxiety were associated in the sample, the association was not due to shared genetic risk but to shared environmental factors that increase the risk of people with dyslexia experiencing anxiety problems such as GAD and panic disorder. Mugnaini et al. (2009) showed that other internalizing disorders such as depression are also common in children with dyslexia. The current evidence therefore suggests that the presence of specific learning disorders such as dyslexia leads to problems in educational and other settings; these in turn are likely to affect the child's self-esteem and lead to an increased risk of internalizing disorders such as depression and anxiety, which are likely to exacerbate the consequences of the disorder.

The acquired language disorders range across the aphasias, aphonias, dysphonias, alexias, and dyslexias, and reflect an acquired impairment to any aspect of previously normal functioning of speech or language. The evidence to date from studies of people with brain damage shows a range of potentially dissociable systems that underlie the different types of language processes, such that deficits can occur specifically to speech comprehension, speech production, reading comprehension, writing, and so on. Aphasia typically results from head injury or stroke and refers to a variety of language disorders that include difficulty with vocabulary, loss of speech, and loss of language comprehension. There has continued to be considerable interest in the neuroanatomical basis for language ever since the classic case studies by Broca and Wernicke in the nineteenth century which identified localized areas of the brain thought to be responsible for language expression and language comprehension. Recent research on the functional neuroanatomy of aphasia suggests that there is a dorsal stream that is involved in the mapping of sound to articulation and a ventral stream in which sound is mapped to meaning, a proposal supported, for example, in a recent MRI study by Kummerer et al. (2013) of 100 patients with acute aphasia.

Disorders of Motor Control

Similar to the disorders of language and memory, there tends to be a greater focus on motor control disorders that either have a neurodevelopmental origin or are acquired because of neurocognitive impairment later in life. However, there is also a category of somatic symptom or conversion disorder problems with motor control that are summarized in classification systems such as DSM-5. Freud (e.g., in Breuer and Freud, 1895) argued that symptoms of hysteria involving motor problems such as paralysis of the limbs originated in the repression of conflictual material that was then expressed by physical means. By contrast, Janet (e.g., Janet, 1920) argued in favor of a *dissociative* origin of such problems rather than them being a consequence of repression. Aspects of both mechanisms have received some, albeit mixed, support in the century or so since their proposal. For example, Kanaan et al. (2007) studied a 37-year-old woman with an unexplained right-sided paralysis that the authors considered was related to a repressed life event—she reported no emotion about her partner's announcement that he was leaving her, an announcement that occurred shortly before the development of her paralysis. The authors nevertheless found high activation of the amygdala on fMRI and concluded that the scanning technique could be used to test such hypotheses concerning repressed emotions about an event. Roelofs et al. (2002) compared a group of 54 patients with a conversion disorder with a matched group of controls with affective disorder on a variety of measures of childhood abuse and current symptoms of dissociation. The conversion disorder group were found to be significantly more likely to have experienced childhood physical or sexual abuse, and maternal dysfunction was associated with higher dissociation scores.

In sum, although there are a wide range of neurodevelopmental and acquired neurocognitive impairments in motor control, and the functional motor conversion disorders now receive less interest than they did in the time of Freud, Charcot, and Janet, there is nevertheless still a category of medically unexplained symptoms in which psychogenic motor control problems arise. Of course, many of these are preceded by an experience of childhood trauma which may be reactivated later by adult life events, and therefore the contribution of emotion is crucial (see Chapter 6). Nevertheless, such disorders further illustrate why it is necessary to consider the joint contribution of drives, emotion, and cognition in the manner that we have emphasized throughout this book.

Conclusions

We have argued that the best starting point for consideration of the cognitive disorders is the underlying cognitive systems on which cognitive and other processes are based. A very straightforward approach to such systems is to consider the basics of perception/attention, thinking/reasoning, memory, language, and motor control, which serendipitously totals a magic five systems akin to the five basic emotion systems that we considered earlier. In this chapter, we have focused primarily on the functional disorders of these cognitive systems, while also noting in passing the range of organic impairments that can occur. The putative cognitive disorders of perception/attention that have been subsumed under the heading of "schizophrenia" do not offer a theoretically consistent grouping of symptoms, in that under current classification systems such as DSM-5 symptoms that originate in perceptual/attentional systems are included alongside symptoms that originate in thinking/reasoning systems. That is, "schizophrenia" can be defined either as a perceptual/attentional disorder or as a thinking/reasoning disorder, which makes no sense from a cognitive systems point of view. If these conflated systems are disentangled from each other, then "schizophrenia" must be divided into at least two disorders, one of which is primarily hallucination-based, so-called hallucinatory disorder, and the second of which is primarily delusion-based, so-called delusional disorder. In fact, it is possible that a further "thought disorder" syndrome may also be extractable from the umbrella category of "schizophrenia," though a variety of different mental states and disorders can give rise to apparent thought disorder.

A second area of some controversy within the cognitive disorders is in relation to memory, in particular the debates in recent years about false memories and repressed memories. Although some people have taken up extreme positions on these aspects of memory, it seems likely that there is some truth in all viewpoints given the constructive and reconstructive nature of memory.

Finally, we need to return to the issue of "belief," one of the fundamental drivers of the cognitive system. The "normal" range of belief and belief systems is considerable, and for every so-called delusional belief held by an individual there is probably a group of people somewhere who may be brought together and united by a similar such "delusional belief." The example was given of the Heaven's Gate Movement, formed by Marshall Applewhite after his NDE, in which the majority of the men castrated themselves and then all members committed suicide, in the belief that they would be taken on board a mothership and transported to an evolutionary level above human. Extreme beliefs are therefore part and parcel of being human, rather than being in and of themselves "disorders." It may be more important to consider how fixed or rigid the belief or belief system is, in terms of whether or not there is some insight into the possibility that the belief system might be wrong and that alternative beliefs are possible. Such an approach emphasizes the value of dimensional approaches to beliefs and other experiential phenomena such as hallucinations rather than seeing such phenomena as qualitatively different to the range of possible normal experiences.

8

OVERVIEW AND IMPLICATIONS

The harder the conflict, the more glorious the triumph

Thomas Paine

Introduction

The history of psychiatry is replete with incorrect theories about the origins and causes of psychological disorders. In Chapter 1 we saw how the most successful theory to date, if we measure success by the length of time for which the theory was influential, was the doctrine of the four humors. Indeed, remnants of the doctrine remain with us today in some of the terms that are used to describe personality types. The theory did not simply provide a model for understanding mental and physical health and ill-health; like any good theory that should also be evaluated in terms of its Popperian usefulness and testability it led to a vast and complex set of practices based on the idea that in illness the four humors of the blood are out of balance and treatments must regain a balance between them. The most common form of treatment was therefore bloodletting. For example, in *The Anatomy of Melancholy* Robert Burton (1621) frequently refers to the different types and uses of bloodletting such as in the treatment of "love-melancholy" which makes "lovers to come to themselves and keep in their right minds" [part 3, p. 194]. The downside of bloodletting as a treatment was clearly that more patients died than were cured, though the mnemonic biases that allow us to forget our mistakes and better remember our successes clearly helped the poor doctors continue their bloodletting practices until something better came along.

An interesting variant on the doctrine of the four humors arose from at least the time of Descartes onwards in which the nerves were thought to be tubes down which a fluid passed causing the muscles to react as in reflex responses. However, because the tubes were very fine, the fluid was thought to be easily blocked and so needed "shock treatment" in order to start flowing again. Like with the humors and bloodletting, this theory led to a whole variety of treatments or cures, some of which were

185

extremely innovative and others incredibly punitive. To walk over an innocent looking bridge that suddenly collapsed and doused people in cold water sounds innovative, whereas "shock" treatment involving beatings with sticks sounds like an excuse
for sadism (e.g., Jones, 1983). The theory of fluid in nerve tubes was eventually shown
to be wrong, though "shock treatments" continue to be used in psychiatry to this day.

The nineteenth century witnessed the rise of the sciences of biology, chemistry,
and physics, and great advances were achieved in each of these disciplines in terms of
our understanding of the mechanics of the universe. Within this context of scientific
excitement and advance, the medicine of the mad turned to biology and chemistry
in order to find a new understanding of madness. German psychiatry, especially in
the unique way that it combined the clinic and the research institute, led the way in
the new science of madness with notable successes, for example Alois Alzheimer's
identification of the deteriorating disease that is most prevalent in old age and that has
now been named after him. Other great German psychiatrists such as Kraepelin and
Bleuler (the latter more correctly being Swiss German) believed that similar advances
could be made with disorders of younger onset such as the disorder that Kraepelin
labeled dementia praecox and Bleuler later renamed schizophrenia. This biological
tradition is of course well represented in our modern approaches to psychiatry and
psychiatric diagnosis, but the problem is that, as we will consider later, psychiatry is
still primarily reliant on symptoms reported by patients rather than on biological
signs that are independent of the patient's self-report. Since Alzheimer's success in
spotting the plaques and other characteristics of Alzheimer's dementia in the early
1900s, and despite the dominance of the biological approach, psychiatry has failed
to make the great steps toward biological understanding that the nineteenth century
seemed to promise. These problems are no more evident than in the mess that has
been created by the current classification and diagnostic systems.

Classification and Diagnosis

We saw in Chapter 2 how in the eighteenth and nineteenth centuries scientists made
great advances in the development of classification systems in biology and chemistry.
By the 1860s 56 different chemical elements were already known when Mendeleev
began work on the periodic table. Mendeleev's theoretical foundation for his classification system was based on the measured atomic weight (then defined as the weight
relative to hydrogen of one mole of the element) of an element, even though this
approach led to some anomalies within the system. Only in the twentieth century,
when the structure of the atom had been identified, was the basis of the classification
system switched to the atomic *number* (the number of protons in the atom) rather

than the atomic weight; this then explained the reason for the anomalies because some elements have two or more isotopes, defined by the number of neutrons rather than protons. In biology, classification systems began a little earlier with the work of Carl Linnaeus, the great Swedish botanist and scientist, in the eighteenth century. Linnaeus based his plant and animal taxonomies on an assessment of the shared physical characteristics and physical differences which were then grouped into hierarchies that captured these physical similarities and differences. The initial Linnaean classification systems were therefore descriptive, but with developments in biology, such as Charles Darwin's theory of evolution, taxonomies based on phylogeny (an organism's evolutionary descent) have been developed, as have more recent systems based on molecular phylogenetics that are largely concerned with the relationships between DNA sequences. However, the moral story to draw from chemistry and biology is that if you want to get ahead, you need to get a theory.

The initial attempts at classification in medicine originated in the work of Farr and D'Espine, who in 1853 had been asked by the International Statistical Congress to produce an agreed list of the causes of death, known as the International List of Causes of Death. From the founding of the World Health Organization in 1948, the ICD as it was known was expanded to include all known diseases, not simply the causes of death, along with a range of psychiatric disorders. Whereas the ICD was therefore designed simply to facilitate the recording of data on illness and death, the DSM, first published in 1952, had a different aim—primarily an attempt to provide "working definitions or thumbnail descriptions of the syndromes concerned" (Kendell, 1975, p. 92). In the first edition of 1952, the DSM was largely influenced by psychoanalytic thinking and the manual included a number of vaguely defined or subsequently controversial categories such as "homosexuality," which in psychoanalytic terms involves fixation at an early psychosexual stage of development plus a set of unresolved unconscious conflicts (see Chapter 2). However, DSM-III, published in 1980, set out under the chairmanship of Robert Spitzer to increase diagnostic reliability through the specification of diagnostic criteria; thus, previous editions of DSM and ICD assumed that clinicians and researchers simply knew from their experience what these criteria were. As any decent psychometrician will tell you, you can't have validity without reliability, and the poor performance of many of the DSM-I and DSM-II categories had been highly problematic. The problem, however, from DSM-III onwards is that just because you have reliability for your diagnostic categories it does not mean you have validity. For example, let us create the "unicorn syndrome" according to the following diagnostic criteria:

belief in a previous existence
feelings of anxiety

episodes of pain in the forehead

wish to dress as, or actually dressing as, a white horse-like creature

significant impact of the condition on work and other social functioning.

Now these five criteria could be very reliably administered using the Fabled Animal Syndrome Taxonomy Version 1 (the FAST-1), such that all psychiatrists on all occasions agreed on the occurrence of a case of unicorn syndrome. The problem, however, is that although the diagnosis may have perfect reliability, it has absolutely no validity.

While Robert Spitzer's attempt to improve the reliability of the DSM system, beginning with DSM-III, was commendable, unfortunately the atheoretical approach to classification used by the developers of the DSM (i.e., based on expert consensus) is fundamentally flawed. Part of the problem with such an approach is that there are obvious risks within a consensus system, including the personal and political factors that lead to certain people being invited to participate and others being excluded from the consensus process, horse-trading around "I'll vote for your favorite category, if you'll vote for mine," and the excessive influence of the powerful individuals who shout the loudest. Richard McNally in *What is Mental Illness?* (McNally, 2011) provides an entertaining account of what goes on behind the scenes at DSM committees, based in part on his own experience, with another insider's view being presented by Allen Frances (2013). Perhaps the most worrying influence behind the scenes is that of the pharmaceutical companies, the world's most profitable multinationals. As McNally summarized:

> Every member of the DSM-IV committees on schizophrenia and mood disorders had financial ties to the pharmaceutical industry, and more than half of those working on the remaining disorders had similarly compromising ties. (McNally, 2011, pp. 35–36)

The financial consequences of eliminating the diagnosis of "schizophrenia" on theoretical grounds could therefore be huge for the pharmaceutical industry, with many of their most profitable products no longer having a target diagnostic category.

The $64,000 question for psychiatric diagnosis is what could provide a theoretical basis for such a system? The success and usefulness of classification systems in biology and chemistry have not been because they got the correct theoretical basis for classification from the outset, but because the anomalies that arose from the classification sometimes provided science with significant questions that prompted further research and advance. For example, the misclassification of iodine and tellurium if arranged by atomic weight was later resolved when the structure of the atom was better understood and the classification system was changed to being based on atomic number rather than atomic weight. Similarly, Mendeleev identified gaps in the periodic table for elements that had not been discovered at that time (the 1860s) but which have been found since. Therefore one of the consequences of using a theoretically based approach to psychiatric classification and diagnosis is that it is likely to cut through current classification categories and slice them up very differently.

Alternatives to Classification and Diagnosis

The clear and pervasive problems with the psychiatric diagnostic and classification systems have led some critics and professional groups to argue that such systems should be abandoned and alternatives used in their place. The first putative alternative that we considered in Chapter 2 was the case formulation approach. Case formulation provides a possible model or theory about an individual's psychological problems in relation to key points of their history, likely causes and precipitants of the problems, maintenance factors that perpetuate the problems, plus some summary of additional vulnerability and resilience factors, but all of this account is framed in terms of a particular theoretical approach (see, e.g., Johnstone and Dallos, 2013, for a useful recent summary). Case formulation brings in theory to the extent that approaches such as behavior therapy, cognitive therapy, or family systems provide an account of the range of psychological disorders. However, as we argued in Chapter 2, when approaches such as behavior therapy or cognitive therapy are examined, they appear to offer nothing better than folk psychology and use terms such as "anxiety," "depression," "eating disorder," or whatever in an ill-defined and loose fashion. That is, although one might argue that the theories of learning that underpin behavior therapy or the theory underlying cognitive therapy have proven themselves invaluable and have made significant contributions both to our understanding of some psychological disorders and to the interventions used to treat some disorders, they do not offer clear explicit theories about what those disorders are or how they relate to each other (Power and Dalgleish, 2008). Our argument therefore is that case formulation, although extremely useful in that it forces clinicians to make explicit the links between their theoretical model, an individual case history, and a proposed intervention for that individual, does not provide an alternative to classification and diagnosis but simply tries to ignore them. However, ignoring the question does not make it go away.

A second alternative, also considered in Chapter 2, is that developed by Mike Berger in his proposal that the World Health Organization's International Classification of Functioning Disability and Health (ICF) (World Health Organization, 2001) could also provide an alternative to the existing diagnostic and classification systems (e.g., Berger, 2008). Again, however, the ICF seems to have the same relationship to classification and diagnosis as does case formulation. That is, the ICF does not provide an alternative to diagnosis, but rather spells out a range of personal and environmental factors that can impact on a possible diagnosis that then determines the level of functioning of the individual with the diagnosis. For example, if you have a diagnosis of short-sightedness (myopia) which is uncorrected, this disorder could lead to disability and poor functioning because the individual is unable to see things clearly at a particular distance. However, the use of an environmental aid (a pair of spectacles) could correct the disability (myopia) and in fact give the individual a better level of functioning than average because the environmental aid provides a perfect correction for the disorder. Therefore the level of functioning within the ICF system is determined by the interaction of a disorder with a range of personal and environmental factors. The ICF system builds on but does not replace the diagnosis and classification systems.

In summary, case formulation and the ICF approach are both highly commendable for the increased understanding that they can bring to our understanding of impairment, disability, and consequent interventions. But they sit alongside, rather than replace, the diagnostic and classification systems.

Theoretical Approaches to Classification—Preliminary Points

In the Preface to this book we raised a number of issues that have an impact on the definition of madness, to which we should now return. These issues are summarized here into three categories in the form of a Venn diagram (see Figure 8.1):

1. Objective madness—madness defined by a set of biological and psychological signs and symptoms according to an agreed classification and diagnostic system.
2. Subjective madness—the individual's personal belief or viewpoint that he or she is suffering from "madness."
3. Socially constructed madness—a social consensus or construction that certain beliefs and actions constitute "madness."

As we noted in the Preface, categories (2) and (3) are in fact more closely related than they seem, in that there is a "constructivist realist" position that is a dominant approach in cognitive psychology (e.g., Neisser, 1976) and in which the individual is seen to create dynamically constructed models of the world that are continually updated. Therefore, although social constructionists (see, e.g., Gergen, 2009) focus on constructionist processes within social relationships, especially as represented in language, there is no inherent contradiction in seeing such processes at work at

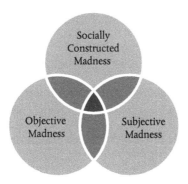

Fig. 8.1. A Venn diagram for the construction of madness.

an intrapsychic level as well as at the interpersonal one. We therefore propose that categories (2) and (3) are closely related variants that arise from the same psychosocial processes. The crucial question for diagnostic systems is therefore that of the potential opposition between "objective" and "constructivist" viewpoints, but with the caveat about levels of constructivism.

In Figure 8.1 the area where all three circles overlap therefore constitutes common ground with all three approaches and includes objective definition, subjective agreement (which might therefore be labeled as "insight"), and social agreement pointing to "madness." By contrast, there are areas where objective and socially constructed madness overlap but subjective madness does not, which could be labeled as "lack of insight"; and an area where subjective and objective madness overlap but socially constructed madness does not, and which could represent, for example, the arguments against the existence of "schizophrenia" as a valid concept.

The Venn diagram in Figure 8.1 summarizes what could be taken as two extreme viewpoints on the definition of madness. First, there is an "all-inclusive" definition which states that the total area covered by the three circles should be included in the definition, that is, even areas where there is no overlap between objective, subjective, or socially constructed. This definition would include cases that were noted in the Preface along the lines of

Sergei believes that he is mad, but nobody else does (society, psychiatry . . .).

Indeed, as we saw in Chapter 6, such an example could be the experience of a single panic attack, which does not meet any diagnostic or other criteria for madness but which nevertheless the individual could experience as "madness" because of a loss of control. The next example, Tom, can simply represent, as noted, a lack of insight into a disorder:

> Tom believes himself not to be mad, but others do (society, psychiatry . . .).

Perhaps the most interesting or most problematic example for the "all-inclusive" definition is socially constructed "madness" in the absence of the subjective or objective:

> Jane believes that she is not mad, psychiatry believes that she is not mad, but society believes that she is mad.

The best examples of such socially constructed madness in the absence of the objective or subjective are the politically motivated categories of "sluggish" or "creeping" schizophrenia that were invented during the Soviet era in order to label as mad some of the critics of the political system. There was of course pressure exerted on Soviet psychiatrists to add such a category into their diagnostic system, but psychiatry more generally opposed such a politically motivated category. Nevertheless, the "all-inclusive" definition of madness—and to be consistent with the acceptance of a subjective state of madness—should include such controversial examples, because they often reflect dynamic reconceptualization processes at a social point in time, as "disorders" become socially defined as, or not defined as, "madness."

The second extreme viewpoint on madness is that in which only the area where all three circles in the Venn diagram overlap counts as "madness," that is, where objective, subjective, and socially constructed madness coincide. However, this "narrow definition" already excludes one of psychiatry's favorite categories in which there is a "lack of insight" into a disorder that the individual has, which may even be denied by the individual. Psychiatry, used here as short-hand to mean those people who support the current classification and diagnostic systems, would therefore definitely want to extend the narrow definition to include the area where the objective and the socially constructed overlap. However, they would probably be jumping up and down about that part of the category of "objective" that does not overlap with subjective or social and why they could not include *all* such cases as well. Again, the reader might ask for an example of an "objective only" category: a powerful example of this would be "homosexuality," which as we saw in Chapter 2 was included as a disorder until DSM-III when social pressures led to its exclusion as a diagnostic category.

An alternative definition to the two extremes that we have considered would be a "middle definition" in which, for example, we might require that at least two out of three of the objective, subjective, and socially constructed viewpoints needed to coincide in order to define "madness." Such a definition would be based on a "majority report" approach. This middle definition would have the advantage of covering the "lack of insight" examples that we have noted, and it could include the subjective examples such as panic attack by a somewhat disingenuous suggestion that there would be at least a subgroup of people who would agree to work with such an experience as a type of madness. However, one of the consequences would be that none of the stand-alone categories, in which there was no overlap with any other category, would by this definition be defined as madness.

Overall, the Venn diagram in Figure 8.1 has served a useful purpose in terms of our deconstruction of possible definitions of madness. At one extreme there is the all-inclusive definition in which madness is that which is defined by at least one of the objective, subjective, or social systems; at the other extreme there is the narrow definition in which all three systems must coincide. Our view throughout this book has tended more toward the middle definition "majority report," in which there is some constructive process (whether it be subjective or social) alongside the objective symptoms, but the objective symptoms in themselves without a subjective and/or social construction would not be sufficient in and of themselves to define madness. This is because psychiatry is a branch of psychology in that it works with subjective symptoms, rather than a branch of medicine, because of its lack of objective signs.

Finally, we should briefly return to the issue of categories versus dimensions in terms of classification and diagnosis. This issue has troubled the classifiers for some time and continues to remain unresolved, as we saw with the fall-out in the DSM-5 Personality and Personality Disorders Work Group (Emmelkamp and Power, 2012). Although the group had set out with the best of intentions to consider how the traditional personality disorder categories might be mapped onto the "big five" normal personality dimensions, they failed to resolve the issue satisfactorily and several members resigned in protest. As a result, DSM-5 comments on possible combinations for personality disorders and personality dimensions but avoids the problem and hands the baton to the future DSM-6 committee and the current ICD-11 committee.

The failure of the makers of DSM-5 to resolve the category versus dimension issue is not surprising, given that the issue raises complex mathematical and philosophical issues. On the surface, the issue can seem deceptively straightforward. For example the approximately normal distribution of the dimension of IQ (at least when conceptualized as a single general factor referred to as "g"; see Deary, 2001) can be "chopped" at the extremes into categories such as "intellectual disability" at IQ < 70 and "genius" at IQ > 140. In the case of a dimension such as IQ, categories can be defined by extreme scores or a range of scores along the dimension; there is no inherent problem when the starting point is a single dimension and category definitions are agreed in this manner. The problem that arises, however, is first a philosophical one in that the classification systems have tended to approach signs and symptoms as categorical—you either have the sign or symptom or you don't—with the patterns of symptoms considered in the same way—you either have the diagnosis or you don't. The first mathematical simplification with this approach is that the category distributions are assumed to be dichotomous, when polychotomous categories may sometimes be more appropriate, such as in the case of body temperature defined as "normal," "high," or "low." Moreover, combining dichotomous and polychotomous categories to produce complex diagnoses begins to lead to quasi-continuous-type distributions for which ranges of scores can be defined. Further complexity arises from combinations of categories and/or dimensions, in that underlying distributions need not be normal and their combinations may lead to apparent interaction effects at the extremes that might not be predictable from the separate constituent categories or dimensions themselves. We considered such unexpected effects in our discussions in Chapters 3 and 4 of gene–environment interactions, which are extremely topical in modern biology; thus, a supposedly "bad" gene (e.g., difficult temperament) may be disadvantageous in a normal environment but offer some survival advantage in a "bad" environment (e.g., famine or drought). The most positive spin on the dimension versus category approaches to classification and diagnosis is to say that there are exciting times ahead that should allow complex modeling of large empirical datasets of symptoms in which the two approaches can be combined mathematically. However, for now we will continue to use a combined approach as appropriate to the different systems; thus, in the case of "basic emotions," we propose that there are five useful categories of emotions, but that each of these occurs on one or more dimensions that reflect the intensity and other properties of the emotion (Power and Dalgleish, 2008).

A Possible Theoretical Basis for Classification

The possible theoretical basis that we offer for diagnosis and classification is the system that we developed in the 1990s (Power and Dalgleish, 1997) and continue to develop to the present day (Power and Dalgleish, 2008). The system is known as the SPAARS approach (for schematic, propositional, analogical, and associative representation systems) and was originally developed as an approach for understanding emotion and the emotional disorders. Because the emotion system has been best examined and developed in both SPAARS and other cognate systems, we will begin with a brief summary of this approach to emotions, before we go on to consider how in this book we have argued for the extension of the SPAARS approach to include drive and cognitive systems and thereby provide sufficient coverage for the full range of psychological disorders.

Emotion and Emotion Disorders

The SPAARS approach to emotion takes as its starting point the proposal that there are five main basic emotions, in agreement with previous researchers such as Oatley and Johnson-Laird (1987). These basic emotions are anger, anxiety, sadness, happiness, and disgust, as shown in Table 8.1. The table also shows two further aspects of the basic emotion proposal. First, complex emotions, for example contempt, irritation, and aggression, are more complex states that are derivable from the basic emotion of anger. However, and in contrast to Oatley and Johnson-Laird (1987), we also argue that some complex emotions and moods need to be derived from two or more basic emotions, such as the example of "nostalgia" which, although listed next to happiness in Table 8.1, in fact consists of a blend of the two basic emotions of happiness and sadness. We should add that it is clear from an analysis of emotion and emotion disorders, and is relevant to our earlier discussion of why psychiatric classification systems are collections of symptoms rather than collections of signs, that an emotion state such as "panic" would have the same set of signs (biological indicators) if it was experienced as "madness" or as a normal reaction such as "my anxiety." That is, an emotion such as panic can be experienced as either normal or abnormal, with the only distinguishing features between the two being the individual's experience and self-report: the two cannot be distinguished at the biological level, therefore, by extension, psychiatric classification systems have to be based on symptoms rather than signs, as we have noted throughout this book.

Table 8.1 also shows some typical emotional disorders that are associated with each of the basic emotions. For example, there are a number of potential anxiety disorders listed in the table that include panic disorder, GAD, phobias (some types), PTSD (some types), and OCD (some types). Whereas in principle some of these, such as panic disorder and GAD, are derivable from the one basic emotion of anxiety, only

Table 8.1: A summary of basic emotions with examples of complex emotions and emotion disorders.

Basic emotion	Complex emotion	Disorder
Anxiety	Worry	GAD
Sadness	Grief	Depression
Anger	Contempt	Pathological anger
Happiness	Nostalgia	Mania
Disgust	Guilt Shame	OCD (contamination)

some types of phobias, PTSD, and OCD are derivable from *just* the basic emotion of anxiety. Up until DSM-IV all phobias, PTSD, and OCD were listed under the "anxiety disorders" despite the clear heterogeneity of their emotion profiles (see, e.g., Power and Fyvie, 2013, for the emotion profiles of PTSD), but in DSM-5 this heterogeneity was dealt with by offering separate chapters for PTSD and OCD such that they were no longer listed as anxiety disorders. However, the theoretically based approach proposed here, which uses the basic emotions as a starting point, requires a Linnaean-type binomial nomenclature to specify the primary basic emotion plus the disorder such as in disgust-phobia, anxiety-phobia, disgust-OCD, anxiety-OCD, and so on. In addition, some of these phobic and other reactions seem to involve two or more basic emotions, which, when coupled together, may go some way to explain the chronicity with which some of the emotional disorders can present. Depression provides another heterogeneous and complex example for classification systems, in that in current systems one depression may have little or no symptom overlap with another. Within a basic emotions approach, depression is a type of disorder of sadness, typically in combination with the complex emotion of shame (derived from the basic emotion of disgust) (Power and Tarsia, 2007), but with other possible contributions from coupling with anxiety and/or anger. Again, an important empirical question to address is an examination of the possible emotion profiles for depression and what their consequences may be for course and outcome of the disorder. Nevertheless, the binomial nomenclature approach of anxiety-depression, anger-depression, and disgust-depression provides a reminder of the heterogeneity of this disorder together with the need for a classification system drawing on a theoretical base that captures the similarities and differences of the various types of depression.

In the extension of the SPAARS system that we have provided in this book as a possible theoretical basis for classification and diagnosis we have argued that emotion, cognition, and drive systems do not stand alone, but that each disorder may be best described in the form of a drive–emotion–cognition (DEC) profile, given that in any disorder there are typically characteristics in common across the three systems. Our example of a panic attack highlights the need for this combination: panic is an emotion state that may be triggered by a threat to physical or social existence but it also has an important cognitive component which can lead to an interpretation of the panic being madness, death, or anxiety (Clark, 1986). That is, in order for panic to be considered as a panic disorder, it is necessary to provide a DEC profile.

The possible DEC profiles across the basic emotions are presented in Table 8.2, which have been summarized from the more detailed examinations provided in Chapter 6. For each basic emotion, it is possible to have a disorder at three different levels (though for the sake of simplicity the levels have not been shown in Table 8.2);

Table 8.2: Drive–emotion–cognition summary: examples for basic emotions.

Drive	Emotion	Cognition
Survival	Anxiety	Threat
Social Drives	Sadness	Loss
Dominance	Anger	Insult
Attachment	Happiness	Superiority
Survival	Disgust	Repulsion

namely, at the basic level, at a complex level with an emotion derived from the basic emotion, and at a coupled level in which two or more coupled basic emotions combine to lead to the disorder. The anxiety disorders provide a clear view of these three levels, with panic and some phobic reactions representing the basic emotion, conditions such as worry representing complex cognitive elaborations of the basic emotion, and a range of coupled states found in some phobias, some types of PTSD, and so on reflecting the combination of anxiety with other basic emotions. Similar analyses are presented in Table 8.2 for sadness and disgust, though the emotions of anger and happiness have been less well analyzed in the literature and deserve considerable further research.

Drives and Their Disorders

In addition to the emotions and their disorders, it is necessary to consider a set of biological states that are essential for our survival but which can also become the focus of disorder. We have labeled these states as drives: we recognize that the use of the term "drives" was at a peak around the mid twentieth century, although its use has declined with the rise and rise of cognitive psychology and the cognitive sciences. However, as we argued in Chapters 4 and 5, the term provides a useful summary of a set of biological survival themes with which organisms are confronted, though we have found it useful to divide these into two subcategories of biological drives and social drives because of the social nature of *Homo sapiens*.

A DEC analysis of the major biological and social drives is presented in Table 8.3, again in a summary form based on the more detailed analyses shown earlier in Chapters 4 and 5. If we take the example of eating disorders, then we hope that the advantages of the DEC analysis will become evident, in that disordered eating does not simply consist of eating too much or too little but either of these states and their various combinations occur in the context of generated emotions and thinking and

Table 8.3: Drive–emotion–cognition summary: examples for drives.

Drive	Emotion	Cognition
Eating	Disgust	Control
Elimination	Disgust	Control
Sex	Anxiety	Impotence
Sleep	Depression	Withdrawal
Survival	Anxiety	Threat
Social	Sadness	Loss

reasoning at both "high-level" and "low-level" systems as summarized in the SPAARS model (Fox and Goss, 2012; Fox and Power, 2009). In fact, the direction of effect is not just from drive state to emotion state, but emotion states and cognitive states impact on drive states such that in order to understand a disordered drive state, such as in an eating disorder, multiple feedback loops between the drive, emotion, and cognitive systems have to be considered.

Table 8.3 also presents in summary some of the social drives and how they may become disordered. In many ways it is more difficult to specify the social drives than their counterpart biological drives because there has been less examination of the nature and range of our social drives. Furthermore, the social drives are more plastic in terms of development and are therefore likely to be more sensitive to different environment states. The interest in developmental studies has therefore been more in what these environmental conditions are than in how these environmental conditions interact with different innate representations of social drives, the example of the interaction of temperament with attachment style being an important one that we considered in Chapter 5 and that has only recently begun to be examined in developmental research. It will only be when these complex social developmental issues are examined in gene–environment models that we will begin to understand order and disorder for social drives.

Cognition and its Disorders

The cognitive system can be considered as a potentially dissociable set of systems that cover perception and attention, memory, thinking and reasoning, language, and motor control—another example of the magic number five that spans the basic emotions, personality traits, the senses (at least in old money), and cognitive systems in the analyses that we have presented here and elsewhere. This cognitive systems approach has also now been incorporated into DSM-5 as part of the recommended assessment of the neurocognitive disorders, though the disorders themselves have not been classified according to the cognitive systems. Perhaps this step will occur for DSM-6. The example that we focused on for the disorders of cognition presented in Chapter 7 was the disorder of "schizophrenia," a diagnostic category that has been the most disputed for many years for a variety of political, theoretical, and empirical reasons. We argued that based on the cognitive systems approach summarized in Table 8.4 the proposal for schizophrenia conflates two separate cognitive systems, the perception–attention system, which involves hallucination-based symptoms, and the thinking–reasoning system, which involves delusion and thought disorder-based symptoms. On the basis of a cognitive systems analysis "schizophrenia" should be divided into at least two and possibly three separate disorders; namely, a hallucinatory disorder that reflects problems within the perception–attention system, a delusional disorder that reflects problems with extreme beliefs within the thinking–reasoning system, and a possible general thought disorder, though the latter may simply reflect the severity of any disorder through its impact on central executive and related functioning. The fact that there are potentially two separate types of "schizophrenia" that the current diagnostic systems mistakenly and confusingly classify together seems to be based in part on the observation that some people with a more prolonged experience of hallucinations can come to develop delusional beliefs about the origins and meaning of these hallucinations. But hallucinations and delusions are in principle produced by separable cognitive systems and should be treated as such; people can generate delusional beliefs about any type of experience or external situation, so there does not appear to be any privileged status that should be given to delusional beliefs that come to be developed about hallucinatory experiences.

Most of the other well-known disorders of cognition are in fact neurological disorders that impact on one or more of the cognitive systems, such as in the case of the

Table 8.4: Drive–emotion–cognition summary: examples for cognitive systems.

Drive	Emotion	Cognition
Memory system	Sadness (etc.)	Memory problems
Perception/attention system	Anxiety	Perception/attention problems
Thinking/reasoning system	Anxiety	Thinking/reasoning problems
Motor system	Disgust	Motor problems
Language system	Anger	Language problems

dementias. These were briefly discussed in Chapter 7, but they are not a primary focus for potential psychological disorders. Nevertheless, the nature of the cognitive systems means that there are other possible functional disorders, for example of memory, language, or motor control. In the case of memory, we examined the possible disorders that might result from the constructive aspects of memory, as in proposals for "false memory syndrome" and memory repression. The reconstructive nature of memory means that reconstructive errors inevitably occur in its proper functioning, and that excess forgetting of emotion-linked memories through processes such as repression and dissociation, as presented originally in the work of Freud and Janet, can provide a problem for individuals who experience such challenges. Similarly, some people may be more vulnerable or suggestible to the development of false memories, whether their source be internal, as in dream and fantasies, or external from the influence of the media and significant others.

Some Implications

The development of a theoretically based diagnosis and classification system will inevitably have important implications: first, for changes to the possible categories of psychological disorders and, secondly, for their possible treatment. These implications have been best examined in relation to the emotions and emotion disorders because the SPAARS model was initially developed to consider the emotions (Power and Dalgleish, 1997, 2008). In *Emotion-Focused Cognitive Therapy* (Power, 2010) a detailed presentation is given of how evidence-based psychological therapies such as CBT and interpersonal psychotherapy (IPT) need to be expanded to incorporate an explicit focus on emotion and how problems with the experience and expression of specific emotions can be dealt with. Sometimes there is too little emotion, or specific emotions such as anger are avoided or repressed; in such cases the client needs to be helped to experience and express the emotion in constructive ways. Intolerance of certain emotion states because they are experienced as aversive can paradoxically lead to them being experienced more often, as Daniel Wegner (e.g., Wegner, 1994) has reported. Teaching the acceptance of aversive emotion states can often therefore be an important step in psychological therapy (Power, 2010). For other clients there is too much emotion, for example an excess of anxiety that seems to be constantly generated, as in the case of sufferers from GAD. Alternative emotion regulation strategies need to be practiced in such cases so that the person can manage the problematic emotions more successfully.

The use of the basic emotions as a foundation for an analysis of the emotional disorders does, as detailed in Chapter 6, leads to the cake being sliced in a different way in comparison to the atheoretical classification systems. For example, if PTSD is no longer considered as just an anxiety disorder but one that can be based on almost any of the basic emotions, either alone or in combination (Dalgleish and Power, 2004), we could suggest that the clinical guideline recommendations (e.g., National Institute for Health and Care Excellence, 2005) that PTSD should be treated with some form of trauma-focused CBT that includes exposure might work well for anxiety-based PTSD but not for anger-based PTSD, which might in fact be exacerbated by exposure-based treatment (Power and Fyvie, 2013). Similar implications should apply to other disorders such as phobias and OCD that have also been treated primarily as anxiety disorders within the classification systems and for which exposure-based CBT treatments are therefore recommended. However, more careful analyses of existing datasets and future outcome studies that examine emotion profiles in such disorders may, as with PTSD, find that the exposure-based treatments work best with the anxiety-based disorders but not necessarily with some of the other emotion states. Again, the standard cognitive behavioral methods including exposure, response prevention, behavioral experiments, cognitive challenge, cognitive acceptance, and so on, will each need to be examined for how they best work with specific emotions.

One of the exciting developments emerging from the SPAARS model has been the role of possible coupling of emotions in the onset and maintenance of psychological disorders. Studies of self-report of emotions have shown, for example, the importance of the emotions of sadness and shame in depression (Power and Tarsia, 2007), and an adaptation of the emotion priming task has shown in a more experimental manner the possible coupling of disgust and anger in eating disorders such as bulimia (Fox and Harrison, 2008) and anorexia (Fox et al., 2013). Although these preliminary findings on emotion coupling need both replication and extension to other emotion disorders, the existence of coupling as a process that is important in the onset and maintenance of emotion disorders means that techniques need to be developed for the *decoupling* of such emotions. The last few years have seen the development of a number of so-called cognitive bias modification (CBM) techniques (e.g., Macleod et al., 2009) that have been developed with a focus on cognitive biases in anxiety and depression. These techniques can be used to train increases or decreases in attentional, memory, and other biases, and the studies to date have offered interesting experimental support for the role that cognitive biases may play in the onset and maintenance of disorders of depression and anxiety. The techniques are in the relatively early days of development and are not just restricted to the use of verbal materials—facial stimuli can also be used (Schmidt et al., 2009)—and they can be extended beyond the anxiety and depression disorders (MacLeod et al., 2009). One interesting possibility therefore is that the CBM techniques can be adapted to demonstrate both coupling and decoupling of emotions in non-clinical populations and across a range of disorders.

The purpose of this section has been to offer just a flavor of the potential implications that the development of a theoretically based classification system could have for research and clinical intervention. There are undoubtedly many other aspects that could be developed, for example pharmacotherapy with the introduction of drugs that could target specific basic emotions and that offer further possibilities for cognitive enhancement in the cognitive disorders. The development of Viagra for the treatment of sexual dysfunction offers such an example of a drug targeted to a specific drive or basic emotion. Viagra (sildenafil citrate) was developed by Pfizer in its UK laboratory in Sandwich, Kent, the original intention being to use it for the treatment of hypertension or angina. However, the preliminary clinical trials revealed that it caused significant penile erections, so Pfizer launched the drug in 1998, marketing it for the treatment of erectile dysfunction. With millions of users worldwide, Viagra and its derivatives have had the interesting side effect of reducing the use of the psychological sex therapies even though the evidence points to best outcomes from the two combined (e.g., Berry, 2013). Nevertheless, the pharmaceutical industry will undoubtedly continue to search for and find "magic bullets" as potent as Viagra for a range of drive, emotion, and cognitive disorders.

Summary and Conclusions

In this book we have presented an overview and critique of modern approaches to psychiatric diagnosis, which, while acknowledging issues such as the reliability and validity of diagnosis, have deliberately remained atheoretical and based on a process of consensus reached by committees. The history of psychiatry is both complex and controversial, and the consensus approach to classification and diagnosis continues to fuel controversy into the modern age. Some critics argue that because consensus is inherently flawed as a procedure, and therefore will constantly be updated according to whim and idiosyncrasy, diagnosis and classification should be abandoned altogether and replaced, for example, with individual case formulation. However, the sciences of biology and chemistry provide examples in which classification systems based on theoretical principles have provided powerful and important levels of understanding. Our argument is therefore that rather than abandon classification and diagnosis in psychiatry and psychology, a better way forward is to develop a theoretical basis for these procedures. We have adapted our own SPAARS approach (Power and Dalgleish, 1997, 2008) that was originally developed to consider emotion and the emotional disorders in a way that makes some headway, we believe, toward the provision of such a theoretical basis through its extension to incorporate social and biological drives and cognitive systems. If such an approach at least points in the direction toward a theoretical basis for diagnosis and classification then we will be grateful, ever mindful that even the great Dmitri Mendeleev did not get the theory behind the periodic table of the elements quite right—only later was the correct basis found. Even if we have only made a fraction of progress in the right direction, this would be one small but important step for our understanding of psychological disorders.

REFERENCES

Abel, E.L. and Sokol, R.J. (1987). Incidence of fetal alcohol syndrome and economic impact of FAS-related anomalies. *Drug and Alcohol Dependence*, 19, 51–70.

Abramson, L.Y., Seligman, M.E.P., and Teasdale, J.D. (1978). Learned helplessness in humans: Critique and reformulation. *Journal of Abnormal Psychology*, 87, 49–74.

Ainsworth, M.D.S., Blehar, M.C., Waters, E., and Wall, S. (1978). *Patterns of Attachment: A Psychological Study of the Strange Situation*. Hillsdale, NJ: Erlbaum.

Alloy, L.B., Abramson, L.Y., Safford, S.M., and Gibb, B.E. (2006). The cognitive vulnerability to depression (CVD) project: Current findings and future directions. In L.B. Alloy and J.H. Riskind (eds.), *Cognitive Vulnerability to Emotional Disorders*, pp. 33–62. Mahwah, NJ: Erlbaum.

American Psychiatric Association (1952). *Diagnostic and Statistical Manual of Mental Disorders* (1st edn.). Washington, DC: American Psychiatric Association.

American Psychiatric Association (1968). *Diagnostic and Statistical Manual of Mental Disorders* (2nd edn.). Washington, DC: American Psychiatric Association.

American Psychiatric Association (1980). *Diagnostic and Statistical Manual of Mental Disorders* (3rd edn.). Washington, DC: American Psychiatric Association.

American Psychiatric Association (1994). *Diagnostic and Statistical Manual of Mental Disorders* (4th edn.). Washington, DC: American Psychiatric Association.

American Psychiatric Association (2013). *Diagnostic and Statistical Manual of Mental Disorders* (5th edn.). Washington, DC: American Psychiatric Association.

Andrews, B. (1995). Bodily shame as a mediator between abusive experiences and depression. *Journal of Abnormal Psychology*, 104, 277–285.

Andrews, B. (1997). Bodily shame in relation to abuse in childhood and bulimia: A preliminary investigation. *British Journal of Clinical Psychology*, 36, 41–50.

Antony, M.M. and Barlow, D.H. (2002). Specific phobias. In D.H. Barlow (ed.), *Anxiety and its Disorders: The Nature and Treatment of Anxiety and Panic*, 2nd edn., pp. 380–417. New York: Guilford.

Averill, J.R. (1982). *Anger and Aggression: An Essay on Emotion*. New York: Springer-Verlag.

Baddeley, A.D. (1996). *Your Memory: A User's Guide*, 3rd edn. London: Prion Books.

Bagshaw, V.E. and McPherson, F.M. (1978). The applicability of the Foulds and Bedford hierarchy model to mania and hypomania. *British Journal of Psychiatry*, 13, 293–295.

Barbui, C., Cipriani, A., Patel, V., Ayuso-Mateos, J.L., and Van Ommeren, M. (2011). Efficacy of antidepressants and benzodiazepines in minor depression: systematic review and meta-analysis. *British Journal of Psychiatry*, 198(Suppl. 1), 11–16.

Barlow, D.H. (ed.) (2002). *Anxiety and its Disorders: The Nature and Treatment of Anxiety and Panic*, 2nd edn. New York: Guilford.

Barnard, P.J. (1993). Modelling users, systems and design spaces. In M.J. Smith and G. Salvendy (eds.), *Human-Computer Interaction Vol. 19: A: Applications and Case Studies. (Advances in Human Factors/Ergonomics)*, pp. 331–336. Amsterdam: Elsevier Science Publishers.

Baron-Cohen, S. (2003). *The Essential Difference*. London: Penguin Books.

Bartholomew, K. (1990). Avoidance of intimacy: An attachment perspective. *Journal of Social and Personal Relationships*, 7, 147–178.

Bartlett, F.C. (1932). *Remembering: A Study in Experimental and Social Psychology*. Cambridge: Cambridge University Press.

Beck, A.T. (1976). *Cognitive Therapy and the Emotional Disorders*. New York: Meridian.

Beck, A.T. and Emery, G. (1985). *Anxiety Disorders and Phobias: A Cognitive Perspective*. New York: Basic Books.

Beck, A.T., Rush, A.J., Shaw, B.F., and Emery, G. (1979). *Cognitive Therapy of Depression: A Treatment Manual*. New York: Guilford Press.

Bentall, R.P. (2009). *Doctoring the Mind: Why Psychiatric Treatments Fail*. London: Penguin Books.

Berger, M. (2008). *A Functional Approach to Clinical Practice: Introducing the International Classification of Functions and its Implications for Clinical Psychology*. Leicester: British Psychological Society.

Berkowitz, L. (1999). Anger. In T. Dalgleish and M.J. Power (eds.), *Handbook of Cognition and Emotion*, pp. 411–428. Chichester: Wiley.

Berrios, G.E. (1995). A history of Parkinson's disease. In G.E. Berrios and R. Porter (eds.), *A History of Clinical Psychiatry*, pp. 95–112. London: Athlone Press.

Berrios, G.E. (1997). The history of mental symptoms: Descriptive psychopathology since the nineteenth century. *Psychological Medicine*, 27, 979–982.

Berry, M. (2013). Sex addiction: The chicken-and-egg dilemma of diagnosis. Opticon1826 (15): 8, doi: <http://dx.doi.org/10.5334/opt.bf>.

Bibring, E. (1953). The mechanism of depression. In P. Greenacre (ed.), *Affective Disorders*, pp. 13–48. New York: International Universities Press.

Blair, J., Mitchell, D., and Blair, K. (2005). *The Psychopath: Emotion and the Brain*. Oxford: Blackwell Publishing.

Booth-LaForce, C. and Oxford, M.L. (2008). Trajectories of social withdrawal from grades 1 to 6: Prediction from early parenting, attachment, and temperament. *Developmental Psychology*, 44, 1298–1313.

Bower, G.H. (1981). Mood and memory. *American Psychologist*, 36, 129–148.

Bowlby, J. (1969). *Attachment and Loss: Vol. 1, Attachment*. London: Hogarth Press.

Bowlby, J. (1980). *Attachment and Loss: Vol. 3, Sadness and Depression*. London: Hogarth Press.

Bowlby, J. (1988). *A Secure Base: Clinical Applications of Attachment Theory*. London: Routledge.

Boyle, M. (2002). *Schizophrenia: A Scientific Delusion*, 2nd edn. London: Routledge.

Boyle, M. (2013). Comment on "Campaign for the Abolition of Schizophrenia Label." *Asylum* (online), <http://www.asylumonline.net/resources/campaign-for-the-abolition-of-schizophrenia-label/>

Breuer, J. and Freud, S. (1895/1974). *Studies on Hysteria* (The Pelican Freud Library, Vol. 3). Harmondsworth: Penguin.

Brewer, W.F. (1974). The problem of meaning and the interrelations of the higher mental processes. In W.B. Weimer and D.S. Palermo (eds.), *Cognition and the Symbolic Processes*, Vol. 1, pp. 263–298. Hillsdale, NJ: Erlbaum.

Brown, G.W., Harris, T.O., and Hepworth, C. (1995). Loss, humiliation and entrapment among women developing depression: A patient and non-patient comparison. *Psychological Medicine*, 25, 7–21.

Bruch, H. (1973). *Eating Disorders: Obesity, Anorexia Nervosa and the Person Within*. London: Routledge and Kegan Paul.

Bruch, H. (1978). *The Golden Cage: The Enigma of Anorexia Nervosa*. Shepton Mallet: Open Books.

Brumariu, L.E. and Sterns, K.A. (2013). Pathways to anxiety: Contributions of attachment history, temperament, peer competence, and ability to manage intense emotions. *Child Psychiatry and Human Development*, 44, 504–515.

Burton, R. (1621/2001). *The Anatomy of Melancholy*. New York: New York Review of Books.

Caspi, A. and Shiner, R. L. (2006). Personality development. In W. Damon and R. Lerner (series eds.) and N. Eisenberg (vol. ed.), *Handbook of Child Psychology, Vol. 3. Social, Emotional, and Personality Development*, 6th edn., pp. 300–365. New York: Wiley.

Caspi, A., Sugden, K., Moffitt, T.E., et al. (2003). Influence of life stress on depression: Moderation by a polymorphism in the 5-HTT gene. *Science*, 301, 386–389.

Cassidy, F. and Carroll, B.J. (2001). The clinical epidemiology of pure and mixed manic episodes. *Bipolar Disorders*, 3, 35–40.

Chaiken, S. and Trope, Y. (1999) (eds.). *Dual-Process Theories in Social Psychology*. New York: Guilford Press.

Champion, L.A. and Power, M.J. (1995). Social and cognitive approaches to depression: Towards a new synthesis. *British Journal of Clinical Psychology*, 34, 485–503.

Chatterji, S. and Bergen, N. (2013). Mood disorders and chronic physical illness. In M.J. Power (ed.), *The Wiley-Blackwell Handbook of Mood Disorders*, 2nd edn. Chichester: Wiley-Blackwell.

Cheung, H.N. and Power, M.J. (2012). The development of a new multidimensional depression assessment scale: Preliminary results. *Clinical Psychology and Psychotherapy*, 19, 170–178.

Chiswick, D. (1998). The relationship between crime and psychiatry. In E.C. Johnstone, C.P.L. Freeman, and A.K. Zealley (eds.), *Companion to Psychiatric Studies*, 6th edn. Edinburgh: Churchill Livingstone.

Cipriani, A., Furukawa, T.A., Salanti, G., et al. (2009). Comparative efficacy and acceptability of 12 new-generation anti-depressants: A multiple-treatments meta-analysis. *The Lancet*, 373, 746–758.

Claridge, G. and Davis, C. (2002). *Personality and Psychological Disorders*. London: Taylor and Francis.

Clark, D.M. (1986). A cognitive approach to panic. *Behaviour Research and Therapy*, 24, 461–470.

Clark, L.A. (2000). Mood, personality, and personality disorder. In R. Davidson (ed.), *Anxiety, Depression, and Emotion*, pp. 171–200. Oxford: Oxford University Press.

Clark, L.A. and Watson, D. (1991). Tripartite model of anxiety and depression: Psychometric evidence and taxonomic implications. *Journal of Abnormal Psychology*, 100, 316–336.

Collerton, D. and Taylor, J.-P. (2013). Advances in the treatment of visual hallucinations in neurodegenerative diseases. *Future Neurology*, 8, 433–444.

Coolidge, F.L. and Segal, D.L. (1998). Evolution of personality disorder diagnosis in the Diagnostic and Statistical Manual of Mental Disorders. *Clinical Psychology Review*, 18, 585–599.

Cooper, J.E., Kendell, R.E., Gurland, B.J., Sharpe, L., Copeland, J.R.M., and Simon, R. (1972). *Psychiatric Diagnosis in New York and London: A Comparative Study of Mental Hospital Admissions*, Maudsley Monographs No. 20. Oxford: Oxford University Press.

Corkin, S. (1968). Acquisition of motor skill after bilateral medial temporal-lobe excision. *Neuropsychologia*, 6, 255–265.

Costa, P.T. Jr. and McCrae, R.R. (1992). *Revised NEO Personality Inventory (NEO-PI-R) and NEO Five-Factor Inventory (NEO-FFI) Professional Manual*. Odessa, FL: Psychological Assessment Resources, Inc.

Craske, M.G. and Waters, A.M. (2005). Panic disorder, phobias, and generalizes anxiety disorder. *Annual Review of Clinical Psychology*, 1, 197–225.

Crick, F. (1994). *The Astonishing Hypothesis: The Scientific Search for the Soul*. New York: Simon and Schuster.

Cronbach, L. (1967). How can instruction be adapted to individual differences. In R. Gagné (ed.), *Learning and Individual Differences*, pp. 23–39. Columbus, OH: Merrill.

Dalgleish, T. and Power, M.J. (2004). Emotion specific and emotion-non-specific components of posttraumatic stress disorder (PTSD): Implications for a taxonomy of related psychopathology. *Behaviour Research and Therapy*, 42, 1069–1088.

Damasio, A. (2005). *Descartes' Error: Emotion, Reason, and the Human Brain*. London: Penguin.

Darwin, C. (1872/1965). *The Expression of the Emotions in Man and Animals*. Chicago, IL: Chicago University Press.

Davidson, R.J. (2000). The functional neuroanatomy of affective style. In R.D. Lane and L. Nadel (eds.), *Cognitive Neuroscience of Emotion*, pp. 371–388. New York: Oxford University Press.

Davies, G.M. and Dalgleish, T. (2001). *Recovered Memories: Seeking the Middle Ground*. Chichester: Wiley.

Dawkins, R. (2006). *The Selfish Gene (30th Anniversary Edition)*. Oxford: Oxford University Press.

Deary, I.J. (2001). *Intelligence: A Very Short Introduction*. Oxford: Oxford University Press.

De Jong, H., Perkins, S., Grover, M., and Schmidt, U. (2011). The prevalence of irritable bowel syndrome in outpatients with bulimia nervosa. *International Journal of Eating Disorders*, 44, 661–664.

De Pauw, S.S. and Mervielde, I. (2010). Temperament, personality and developmental psychopathology: A review based on the conceptual dimensions underlying childhood traits. *Child Psychiatry and Human Development*, 41, 313–329.

Der, G., Gupta, S., and Murray, R. (1990). Is schizophrenia disappearing? *The Lancet*, 335, 513–516.

Descartes, R. (1649/1989). *The Passions of the Soul*. Indianapolis, IN: Hackett.

DeVries, M.W. (1984). Temperament and infant mortality among the Masai of East Africa. *American Journal of Psychiatry*, 141, 1189–1194.

De Waal, F. (1996). *Good Natured*. Harvard, MA: Harvard University Press.

DiGiuseppe, R. and Tafrate, R.C. (2007). *Understanding Anger Disorders*. Oxford: Oxford University Press.

Digman, J.M. (1990). Personality structure: Emergence of the five-factor model. *Annual Review of Psychology*, 41, 417–440.

Dima, A.L., Gillanders, D.T., and Power, M.J. (2013). Dynamic pain-emotion relations in chronic pain: A theoretical review of moderation studies. *Health Psychology Review*, 7, S185–S252.

Domhoff, W. (2003). *The Scientific Study of Dreams: Neural Networks, Cognitive Development, and Content Analysis*. Washington, DC: American Psychological Association.

Eells, T.D. (ed.) (1997). *Handbook of Psychotherapy Case Formulation*. New York: Guilford Press.

Ehlers, A. and Clark, D. (2000). A cognitive model of posttraumatic stress disorder. *Behaviour Research and Therapy*, 38, 319–345.

Ekman, P. (1999). Basic emotions. In T. Dalgleish and M.J. Power (eds.), *Handbook of Cognition and Emotion*, pp. 45–60. Chichester: Wiley.

Ekman, P. (2003). *Emotions Revealed: Understanding Faces and Feelings*. London: Weidenfeld and Nicolson.

Ekman, P. and Davidson, R.J. (eds.) (1994). *The Nature of Emotion: Fundamental Questions*. Oxford: Oxford University Press.

Ellenberger, H. (1970). *The Discovery of the Unconscious: The History and Evolution of Dynamic Psychiatry*. New York: Basic Books.

Ellis, A. and Sagarin, E. (1965). *Nymphomania: A Study of the Oversexed Woman*. New York: MacFadden.

Elsabbagh, M., Mercure, E., Hudry, K., et al. (2012). Infant neural sensitivity to dynamic eye gaze is associated with later emerging autism. *Current Biology*, 22, 338–342.

Emmelkamp, P. and Power, M.J. (2012). DSM-5 personality disorders: Stop before it is too late. *Clinical Psychology and Psychotherapy*, 19, 363.

Eysenck, H.J. (1947). *Dimensions of Personality*. London: Routledge and Kegan Paul.

Eysenck, M.W. (1997). *Anxiety and Cognition: A Unified Theory*. Hove: Psychology Press.

Eysenck, H.J. and Eysenck, M.W. (1985). *Personality and Individual Differences: A Natural Science Approach*. New York: Plenum Press.

Eysenck, M.W. and Keane, M.T. (2010). *Cognitive Psychology: A Student's Handbook*, 6th edn. Hove: Psychology Press.

Fairburn, C.G. (1996). Eating disorders. In D.M. Clark and C.G. Fairburn (eds.), *Science and Practice of Cognitive Behaviour Therapy*, pp. 209–242. Oxford: Oxford University Press.

Fairburn, C.G. and Harrison, P.J. (2003). Eating disorders. *The Lancet*, 361, 407–416.

Fairburn, C.G., Cooper, P.J., and Cooper, Z. (1986). The clinical features and maintenance of bulimia nervosa. In K.D. Brownell and J.P. Foreyt (eds.), *Physiology, Psychology and Treatment of the Eating Disorders*, pp. 389–404. New York: Basic Books.

Fairburn, C.G., Cooper, Z., and Shafran, R. (2003). Cognitive behaviour therapy for eating disorders: A "transdiagnostic" theory and treatment. *Behaviour Research and Therapy*, 41, 509–528.

Fava, M., Anderson, K., and Rosenbaum, J.F. (1993). Are thymoleptic-responsive "anger attacks" a discrete clinical syndrome? *Psychosomatics*, 34, 350–355.

Field, A. (2006). Is conditioning a useful framework for understanding the development and treatment of phobias? *Clinical Psychology Review*, 26, 857–875.

Fine, C. (2010). *Delusions of Gender: The Real Science Behind Sex Differences*. London: Icon Books.

Finkelhor, D. (2008). *Childhood Victimization: Violence, Crime, and Abuse in the Lives of Young People*. Oxford: Oxford University Press.

Finlay-Jones, R., and Brown, G.W. (1981) Types of stressful life event and the onset of anxiety and depressive disorders. *Psychological Medicine*, 11, 803–815.

Foa, E.B. and Rothbaum, B.O. (1998). *Treating the Trauma of Rape: Cognitive-Behavioural Therapy for PTSD*. New York: Guilford.

Fonagy, P., Target, M., and Gergely, G. (2003). The developmental roots of borderline personality disorder in early attachment relationships: A theory and some evidence. *Psychoanalytic Inquiry*, 23, 412–459.

Foucault, M. (1971). *Madness and Civilization: A History of Insanity in the Age of Reason*. London: Tavistock.

Foulds, G.A. (1976). *The Hierarchical Nature of Personal Illness*. New York: Academic Books.

Foulds, G.A. and Bedford, A. (1975). Hierarchy of classes of personal illness. *Psychological Medicine*, 5, 181–192.

Fox, J. and Goss, K. (eds.) (2012). *Eating and its Disorders*. Chichester: Wiley-Blackwell.

Fox, J.R.E. and Harrison, A. (2008). The relation of anger to disgust: The potential role of coupled emotions within eating pathology. *Clinical Psychology and Psychotherapy*, 15, 86–95.

Fox, J.R.E. and Power, M.J. (2009). Eating disorders and multi-level models of emotion: An integrated model. *Clinical Psychology and Psychotherapy*, 16, 240–268.

Fox, J.R.E., Federici, A., and Power, M.J. (2012). Emotions and eating disorders. In J.R.E. Fox and K.P. Goss (eds.), *Eating and its Disorders*, pp. 167–184. Chichester: Wiley-Blackwell.

Fox, J.R.E., Smithson, E., Baillie, S., Ferreira, N., Mayr, I., and Power, M.J. (2013). Emotion coupling and regulation in anorexia nervosa. *Clinical Psychology and Psychotherapy*, 20, 319–333.

Frances, A. (2013). *Saving Normal: An Insider's Revolt Against Out-Of-Control Psychiatric Diagnosis, DSM-5, Big Pharma, and the Medicalization of Ordinary Life*. New York: William Morrow.

Franco, B. (2003). Major depressive disorder with anger: A bipolar spectrum disorder? *Psychotherapy and Psychosomatics*, 72, 300–306.

Frank, J.D. (1973). *Persuasion and Healing: A Comparative Study of Psychotherapy*. New York: Schocken Books.

Franzini, L.R. and Grossberg, J.M. (1995). *Eccentric and Bizarre Behaviors*. New York: Wiley.

Fredrickson, B. (2009). *Positivity: Groundbreaking Research to Release Your Inner Optimist and Thrive*. London: Oneworld.

Freud, S. (1899). Screen memories. In *The Standard Edition of the Complete Psychological Works of Sigmund Freud*, Vol. 3, p. 301. London: Hogarth Press.

Freud, S. (1900). *The Interpretation of Dreams*. London: Hogarth Press.

Freud, S. (1905). Three essays on the theory of sexuality. In *The Standard Edition of the Complete Psychological Works of Sigmund Freud*, Vol. 7, p. 125. London: Hogarth Press.

Freud, S. (1915/1949). The unconscious. In J. Strachey (ed. and transl.) *The Standard Edition of the Complete Psychological Works of Sigmund Freud*, Vol. 14, pp. 159–216. London: Hogarth Press.

Freud, S. (1917/1984). *Mourning and Melancholia*, Pelican Freud Library, Vol. 11. Harmondsworth: Penguin.

Freud, S. (1920/1949). Beyond the pleasure principle. In J. Strachey (ed. and transl.) *The Standard Edition of the Complete Psychological Works of Sigmund Freud*, Vol. 18, pp. 7–66. London: Hogarth Press.

Frommann, I., Pukrop, R., Brinkmeyer, J., et al. (2011). Neuropsychological profiles in different at-risk states of psychosis: Executive control impairment in the early—and additional memory dysfunction in the late—prodromal state. *Schizophrenia Bulletin*, 37, 861–873.

Garety, P.A. and Hemsley, D.R. (1994). *Delusions: Investigation into the Psychology of Delusional Reasoning*. Oxford: Oxford University Press.

Garety, P.A., Kuipers, E., Fowler, D., Freeman, D., and Bebbington, P.E. (2001). A cognitive model of the positive symptoms of psychosis. *Psychological Medicine*, 31, 189–195.

Gay, P. (1988). *Freud: A Life for Our Time*. London: Dent.

Geddes, J.R., Carney, S.M., Davies, C., et al. (2003). Relapse prevention with antidepressant drug treatment in depressive disorders: A systematic review. *The Lancet*, 361, 653–661.

Gergen, K.J. (2009). *An Invitation to Social Construction*, 2nd edn. London: Sage.

Gibbons, R.D., Brown, C.H., Hur, K., Davis, J.M., and Mann, J.J. (2012). Suicidal thoughts and behaviour with antidepressant treatment: Reanalysis of the randomized placebo-controlled studies of fluoxetine and venlafaxine. *Archives of General Psychiatry*, 69, 580–587.

Gilbert, P. (1989). *Human Nature and Suffering*. Hove: Erlbaum.

Gilbert, P. (2004). Depression: A biopsychosocial, integrative, and evolutionary approach. In M.J. Power (ed.), *Mood Disorders: A Handbook of Science and Practice*, pp. 99–142. Chichester: Wiley.

Gilbert, P. (2013). Depression: The challenges of an integrative, biopsychosocial evolutionary approach. In M.J. Power (ed.), *The Wiley-Blackwell Handbook of Mood Disorders*, pp. 229–288. Chichester: Wiley-Blackwell.

Goffman, E. (1961). *Asylums: Essays on the Social Situation of Mental Patients and Other Inmates*. New York: Anchor Books.

Goldberg, D. and Goodyer, I.M. (2005). *The Origins and Course of Common Mental Disorders*. London: Routledge.

Goldstein, A.J. and Chambless, D.L. (1978). A reanalysis of agoraphobia. *Behavior Therapy*, 9, 47–59.

Goodman, L.A., Rosenberg, S.D., Mueser, K.T., et al. (1997). Physical and sexual assault history in women with serious mental illness: Prevalence, correlates, treatment, and future research directions. *Schizophrenia Bulletin*, 23, 685–696.

Goodwin, F.K. and Jamison, K.R. (2007). *Manic-Depressive Illness: Bipolar Disorders and Recurrent Depression*, 2nd edn. Oxford: Oxford University Press.

Gray, J.A. (1982). *The Neuropsychology of Anxiety*. Oxford: Oxford University Press.

Groneman, C. (2000). *Nymphomania: A History*. New York: Norton.

Grunbaum, A. (1984). *The Foundations of Psychoanalysis*. Berkeley, CA: University of California Press.

Gudjonsson, G.H. (2001). *The Psychology of Interrogations and Confessions*. Chichester: Wiley.

Gunduz-Bruce, H., McMeniman, M., Robinson, D.G., et al. (2005). Duration of untreated psychosis and time to treatment response for delusions and hallucinations. *American Journal of Psychiatry*, 162, 1966–1969.

Harlow, H.F. (1959). Love in infant monkeys. *Scientific American*, 68, 72–73.

Harre, R. (1987). *The Social Construction of Emotions*. Oxford: Blackwell.

Harris, C.R. (2003). A review of sex differences in sexual jealousy, including self-report data, psychophysiological responses, interpersonal violence, and morbid jealousy. *Personality and Social Psychology Review*, 7, 102–128.

Harter, S. (1977). A cognitive-developmental approach to children's expression of conflicting feelings and a technique to facilitate such expression in play therapy. *Journal of Consulting and Clinical Psychology*, 45, 417–432.

Harter, S. (1999). *The Construction of the Self: A Developmental Perspective*. New York: Guilford.

Harter, S. and Buddin, B. (1987). Children's understanding of the simultaneity of two emotions: A five-stage developmental acquisition sequence. *Developmental Psychology*, 23, 388–399.

Hazan, C. and Shaver, P. (1987). Romantic love conceptualised as an attachment process. *Journal of Personality and Social Psychology*, 52, 511–524.

Healy, D. (2008). *Mania: A Short History of Bipolar Disorder*. Baltimore, MD: The Johns Hopkins University Press.

Hejl, A., Hogh, P., and Waldemar, G. (2002). Potentially reversible conditions in 1000 consecutive memory clinic patients. *Journal of Neurology, Neurosurgery and Psychiatry*, 73, 390–394.

Hekmat, H. (1987). Origins and development of human fear reactions. *Journal of Anxiety Disorders*, 1, 197–218.

Herman, J.L. (1992). *Trauma and Recovery*. New York: Basic Books.

Hermelin, B. and O'Connor, N. (1970). *Psychological Experiments with Autistic Children*. London: Pergamon Press.

Hilbert, A. and Tuschen-Caffier, B. (2007). Maintenance of binge eating through negative mood: a naturalistic comparison of binge eating disorder and bulimia nervosa. *International Journal of Eating Disorders*, 40, 521–530.

Hirschfeld, R.M.A. and Weissman, M.M. (2002). Risk factors for major depression and bipolar disorder. In K.L. Davis, D. Charney, J.T. Coyle, and C. Nemeroff (eds.), *Neuropsychopharmacology: The Fifth Generation of Progress*, pp. 1017–1025. Philadelphia, PA: Lippincott.

Holmes, D.S. (1990). The evidence for repression: An examination of 60 years of research. In J.L. Singer (ed.), *Repression and Dissociation*. Chicago, IL: University of Chicago Press.

Hull, C.L. (1943). *Principles of Behavior*. New York: Appleton-Century-Crofts.

Humphrey, N. (2008). *The Mind Made Flesh: Essays from the Frontiers of Psychology and Evolution*. Oxford: Oxford University Press.

Hunter, E.M. (2011). Multisensory integration of social information in adult aging. Ph.D Thesis, University of Edinburgh.

Hyun, M., Friedman, S.D., and Dunner, D.L. (2000). Relationship of childhood physical and sexual abuse to adult bipolar disorder. *Bipolar Disorders*, 2, 131–135.

Jackson, S.W. (1986). *Melancholia and Depression: From Hippocratic Times to Modern Times*. New Haven, CT: Yale University Press.

Janet, P. (1889). *L'Automatisme Psychologique: Essai de Psychologie Mentale sur les Formes Inferieures de l'activite Mentale*. Paris: Alcan.

Janet, P. (1920). *The Major Symptoms of Hysteria*, 2nd edn. London: Macmillan.

Jansen, A., Havermans, R., Nederkoorn, C., and Roefs, A. (2008). Jolly fat or sad fat? Subtyping non-eating disordered overweight and obesity along an affect dimension. *Appetite*, 51, 635–640.

Jauhar, S. and Cavanagh, J. (2013). Classification and epidemiology of bipolar disorder. In M.J. Power (ed.), *The Wiley-Blackwell Handbook of Mood Disorders*, 2nd edn., pp. 291–309. Chichester: Wiley-Blackwell.

Johnson-Laird, P.N. and Oatley, K. (1989). The language of emotions: An analysis of a semantic field. *Cognition and Emotion*, 3, 81–123.

Johnstone, L. and Dallos, R. (2013). *Formulation in Psychology and Psychotherapy: Making Sense of People's Problems*, 2nd edn. London: Routledge.

Johnstone, E.C., Deakin, J.F.W., Lawlor, P., et al. (1980). The Northwick Park ECT trial. *The Lancet*, ii, 1317–1320.

Jones, W.L. (1983). *Ministering to Minds Diseased: A History of Psychiatric Treatment*. London: Heinemann.

Jowett, B. (transl.) (1953). *The Timaeus* [Plato]. Oxford: Oxford University Press.

Juhasz, G., Dunham, J.S., McKie, S., et al. (2011). The CREB1-BDNF-NTRK2 pathway in depression: Multiple gene-cognition-environment interactions in depression. *Biological Psychiatry*, 69, 762–771.

Kagan, J. (1998). *Galen's Prophecy: Temperament in Human Nature*. New York: Westview Press.

Kahneman, D. (2011). *Thinking Fast and Slow*. London: Allen Lane.

Kanaan, R.A.A., Craig, T.K.J., Wesseley, S.C., and David, A.S. (2007). Imaging repressed memories in motor conversion disorder. *Psychosomatic Medicine*, 69, 202–205.

Karg, K., Burmeister, M., Shedden, K., and Sen, S. (2011). The serotonin transporter promoter variant (5-HTTLPR), stress, and depression meta-analysis revisited: Evidence of genetic moderation. *Archives of General Psychiatry*, 68, 444–454.

Kempe, M. (2004). *The Book of Margery Kempe*. London: Penguin.

Kendell, R.E. (1975). The concept of disease and its implications for psychiatry. *British Journal of Psychiatry*, 127, 305–315.

Kendler, K.S., Hettema, J.H., Butera, F., Gardner, C.O., and Prescott, C.A. (2003). Life event dimensions of loss, humiliation, entrapment, and danger in the prediction of onsets of major depression and generalized anxiety. *Archives of General Psychiatry*, 60, 789–796.

Kendler, K.S. and Shuman, L. (1997). Stressful life events and genetic liability to major depression: Genetic control of exposure to the environment. *Psychological Medicine*, 27, 539–547.

Kendler, K.S., Thornton, L.M., and Gardner, C.O. (2001). Genetic risk, number of previous episodes, and stressful life events in predicting onset of major depression. *American Journal of Psychiatry*, 158, 582–586.

Kennedy A.P., Gask L.L., and Rogers A.E. (2005). Training professionals to engage with and promote self-management. *Health Education Research*, 20, 567–578.

Kesey, K. (1962). *One Flew Over the Cuckoo's Nest*. New York: Viking Press.

Klein, D.F. (1981). Anxiety reconceptualized. In D.F. Klein and J.G. Rabkin (eds.), *Anxiety: New Research and Changing Concepts*, pp. 235–264. New York: Raven Press.

Knowles, G.J. (1999). Male prison rape: A search for causation and prevention. *The Howard Journal of Criminal Justice*, 38, 267–282.

Konstantakopoulos, G., Varsou, E., Ploumpidis, D., et al. (2013). Is there delusional anorexia nervosa? *European Psychiatry*, 28(Suppl. 1), 1.

Kopelman, M. and Morton, J. (2001). Psychogenic amnesias: functional memory loss. In G.M. Davies and T. Dalgleish (eds.), *Recovered Memories: Seeking the Middle Ground*, pp. 219–243. Chichester: Wiley.

Kotov, R., Ruggero, C.J., Krueger, R.F., Watson, D., Yuan, Q., and Zimmerman, M. (2011). New dimensions in the quantitative classification of mental illness. *Archives of General Psychiatry*, 68, 1003–1011.

Kramer, H. and Sprenger, J. (1487/1971). *Malleus Maleficarum*. New York: Dover.

Kummerer, D., Hartwigsen, G., Kellmeyer, P., et al. (2013). Damage to ventral and dorsal language pathways in acute aphasia. *Brain*, 136, 619–629.

Lambek, M. (1981). *Human Spirits: A Cultural Account of Trance in Mayotte*. New York: Cambridge University Press.

Lang, P.J. (1985). The cognitive psychophysiology of emotion: Fear and anxiety. In A.H. Tuma and J.D. Maser (eds.), *Anxiety and the Anxiety Disorders*, pp. 131–170. Hillsdale, NJ: Erlbaum.

Lawrence, C.H. (2001). *Medieval Monasticism: Forms of Religious Life in Western Europe in the Middle Ages*. Harlow: Longman.

Lawton, R. and Nutter, A. (2002). A comparison of reported levels and expression of anger in everyday and driving situations. *British Journal of Psychology*, 93, 407–423.

LeDoux, J.E. (1996). *The Emotional Brain: The Mysterious Underpinnings of Emotional Life*. New York: Simon and Schuster.

Leventhal, H. and Scherer, K. (1987). The relationship of emotion to cognition: A functional approach to a semantic controversy. *Cognition and Emotion*, 1, 3–28.

Lewis-Williams, D. (2010). *Conceiving God: The Cognitive Origin and Evolution of Religion*. London: Thames and Hudson.

Liddle, P.F. (1987). The symptoms of chronic schizophrenia. A re-examination of the positive-negative dichotomy. *British Journal of Psychiatry*, 151, 145–151.

Loftus, E.F. (1998). Imaginary memories. In M.A. Conway, S.E. Gathercole, and C. Cornoldi (Eds.), *Theories of Memory*, Vol. II, pp. 135–145. Hove: Psychology Press.

Loftus, E.F. and Loftus, G.R. (1980). On the permanence of stored information in the human brain. *American Psychologist*, 35, 409–420.

Loftus, E.F. and Pickrell, J.E. (1995). The formation of false memories. *Psychiatric Annals*, 25, 720–725.

Loftus, E. and Zanni, G. (1975). Eyewitness testimony: The influence of the wording of a question. *Bulletin of the Psychonomic Society*, 5, 86–88.

Lutz, C.A. (1988). *Unnatural Emotions: Everyday Sentiments on a Micronesian Atoll and Their Challenge to Western Theory*. Chicago, IL: University of Chicago Press.

McCrae, R.R. and Costa, P.T. (1987). Validation of the five-factor model of personality across instruments and observers. *Journal of Personality and Social Psychology*, 52, 81–90.

McCrory, E., Stephane, A., De Brito, S.A., and Viding, E. (2010). Research review: The neurobiology and genetics of maltreatment and adversity. *Journal of Child Psychology and Psychiatry*, 51, 1079–1095.

McDonald, S. and Flanagan, S. (2004) Social perception deficits after traumatic brain injury: The interaction between emotion recognition, mentalising ability and social communication. *Neuropsychology*, 18, 572–579.

McGorry, P.D. (1994). The influence of illness duration on syndrome clarity and stability in functional psychosis: Does the diagnosis emerge and stabilize with time? *Australian and New Zealand Journal of Psychiatry*, 28, 607–619.

Macleod, C., Koster, E.H., and Fox, E. (2009). Whither cognitive bias modification research? Commentary on the special section articles. *Journal of Abnormal Psychology*, 118, 89–99.

McNally, R.J. (1990). Psychological approaches to panic disorder: A review. *Psychological Bulletin*, 108, 403–419.

McNally, R.J. (2011). *What is Mental Illness?* Harvard, MA: Harvard University Press.

Main, M. and Solomon, J. (1986). Discovery of an insecure-disorganized/disoriented attachment pattern. In T.B. Brazelton and M.W. Yogman (eds.), *Affective Development in Infancy*, pp. 95–124. Westport, CT: Ablex Publishing.

Mancini, F., Gragnani, A., and D'Olimpio, F. (2001). The connection between disgust and obsessions and compulsions in a non-clinical sample. *Personality and Individual Differences*, 31, 1173–1180.

Maslow, A.H. (1954). *Toward a Psychology of Being*. New York: Van Nostrand Reinhold.

Maudsley, H. (1870). *Body and Mind*. New York: Appleton.

Mellers, J.D.C., Sham, P., Jones, P.B., Toone, B.K., and Murray, R.M. (1996). A factor analytic study of symptoms in acute schizophrenia. *Acta Psychiatrica Scandinavica*, 93, 92–98.

Moffitt, T.E., Caspi, A., and Rutter, M. (2006). Measured gene–environment interactions in psychopathology: Concepts, research strategies, and implications for research, intervention, and public understanding of genetics. *Perspectives on Psychological Science*, 1, 5–27.

Morin, C.M. and Espie, C.A. (2003). *Insomnia: A Clinical Guide to Assessment and Treatment*. New York: Springer.

Mowrer, O.H. (1960). *Learning Theory and Behavior*. New York: Wiley.

Mueser, K.T., Drake, R.E., and Noordsy, D.L. (1998). Integrated mental health and substance abuse treatment for severe psychiatric disorders. *Journal of Practical Psychiatry and Behavioral Health*, 4, 129–139.

Mugnaini, D., Lassi, S., La Malfa, G., and Albertini, G. (2009). Internalizing correlates of dyslexia. *World Journal of Pediatrics*, 5, 255–264.

Myers, L.B. and Brewin, C.R. (1994). Recall of early experience and the repressive coping style. *Journal of Abnormal Psychology*, 103, 288–292.

Myers, L.B., Brewin, C.R., and Power, M.J. (1998). Repressive coping and the directed forgetting of emotional material. *Journal of Abnormal Psychology*, 107, 141–148.

Myers, J.K., Weissman, M.M., and Tischler, G.L., et al. (1984). Six-month prevalence of psychiatric disorders in three communities. *Archives of General Psychiatry*, 41, 959–967.

Myhrman, M., Rantakalio, P., Isohanni, M., Jones, P., and Partanen, U. (1996). Unwantedness of a pregnancy and schizophrenia in the child. *British Journal of Psychiatry*, 169, 637–640.

National Institute for Health and Care Excellence (2005). *Depression in Children and Young People*. NICE Clinical Guideline 28. London: National Institute for Health and Care Excellence.

National Institute for Health and Care Excellence (2009). *Depression in Adults*. NICE Clinical Guideline 90. London: National Institute for Health and Care Excellence.

Nederhof, M.J. (2009). *Dispute of a man with his ba*. Available at: <http://mjn.host.cs.st-andrews.ac.uk/egyptian/texts/corpus/pdf/>.

Neisser, U. (1976). *Cognition and Reality*. San Francisco: Freeman.

Newman, L.S. and Baumeister, R.F. (1998). Abducted by aliens: Spurious memories of interplanetary masochism. In S.J. Lynn and K.M. McConkey (eds.), *Truth in Memory*, pp. 282–303. New York: Guilford Press.

Norman, D.A. and Shallice, T. (1980). *Attention to Action: Willed and Automatic Control of Behavior*, CHIP Report 99. San Diego: University of California.

Novaco, R.W. (1979). The cognitive regulation of anger and stress. In P.C. Kendall and S.D. Hollon (eds.), *Cognitive-Behavioural Interventions: Theory, Research, and Procedures*, pp. 241–282. New York: Academic Press.

Novaco, R.W. and Chemtob, C.M. (2002). Anger and combat-related posttraumatic stress disorder. *Journal of Traumatic Stress*, 15, 123–132.

Oatley, K. (2004). *Emotions: A Brief History*. Oxford: Blackwell.

Oatley, K. and Johnson-Laird, P.N. (1987). Towards a cognitive theory of emotions. *Cognition and Emotion*, 1, 29–50.

Ogden, J. (2010). *The Psychology of Eating*, 2nd edn. Chichester: Wiley-Blackwell.

Ohman, A. and Mineka, S. (2001). Fears, phobias, and preparedness: Toward an evolved module of fear and fear learning. *Psychological Review*, 108, 483–522.

Orange, R. (2012). *The Mind of a Madman: Norway's Struggle to Understand Anders Breivik*. Amazon: Kindle Book.

Osgood, C.E., Suci, G.J., and Tannenbaum, P.H. (1957). *The Measurement of Meaning*. Urbana, IL: University of Illinois.

Parkes, C.M. (1993). Bereavement as a psychosocial transition: Processes of adaptation to change. In M.S. Stroebe, W. Stroebe, and R.O. Hansson (eds.), *Handbook of Bereavement: Theory, Research, and Intervention*, pp. 91–101. Cambridge: Cambridge University Press.

Parkes, C.M., Laungani, P., and Young, B. (eds.) (1997). *Death and Bereavement Across Cultures*. London: Routledge.

Paterson, G. and Sanson, A. (1999). The association of behavioural adjustment to temperament, parenting and family characteristics among five-year-old children. *Social Development*, 8, 293–309.

Petersen, R.C. (2004). Mild cognitive impairment as a diagnostic entity. *Journal of Internal Medicine*, 256, 183–194.

Petersen, T., Harley, R., Papkostas, G.I., Montoya, H.D., Fava, M., and Alpert, J.E. (2004). Continuation cognitive-behavioural therapy maintains attributional style improvement in depressed patients responding acutely to fluoxetine. *Psychological Medicine*, 34, 555–561.

Peterson, C., Maier, S.F., and Seligman, M.E.P. (1993). *Learned Helplessness: A Theory for the Age of Personal Control*. New York: Oxford University Press.

Phillips, K.F.V. and Power, M.J. (2007). A new self-report measure of emotion regulation in adolescents: The Regulation of Emotions Questionnaire. *Clinical Psychology and Psychotherapy*, 14, 145–156.

Phillips, M.L., Marks, I.M., Senior, C., et al. (2000). A differential neural response in obsessive-compulsive disorder patients with washing compared with checking symptoms to disgust. *Psychological Medicine*, 30, 1037–1050.

Phillips, K.A., Hart, A.S., Coles, M.E., Eisen, J.L., Menard, W., and Rasmussen, S.A. (2012). A comparison of insight in body dysmorphic disorder and obsessive-compulsive disorder. *Journal of Psychiatric Research*, 46, 1293–1299.

Pilgrim, D. (2009). *Key Concepts in Mental Health*. London: Sage.

Pinker, S. (2011). *The Better Angels of Our Nature*. London: Allen Lane.

Polivy, J. and Herman, C. (2002). Causes of eating disorders. *Annual Review of Psychology*, 53, 187–213.

Popper, K. (1963). *Conjectures and Refutations: The Growth of Scientific Knowledge*. London: Routledge.

Porter, R. (1990). *Mind-Forg'd Manacles: A History of Madness in England from the Restoration to the Regency*. London: Penguin.

Porter, R. (1995). *The Facts of Life: The Creation of Sexual Knowledge in Britain, 1650–1950*. Yale: Yale University Press.

Porter, R. (2002). *Madness: A Brief History*. Oxford: Oxford University Press.

Porter, C.L. (2009). Predicting preschoolers' social-cognitive play behavior: Attachment, peers, temperament, and physiological regulation. *Psychological Reports*, 104, 517–528.

Power, M.J. (1997). Conscious and unconscious representations of meaning. In M.J. Power and C.R. Brewin (eds.), *The Transformation of Meaning in Psychological Therapies*, pp. 57–73. Chichester: Wiley.

Power, M.J. (1999). Sadness and its disorders. In T. Dalgleish and M.J. Power (eds.), *Handbook of Cognition and Emotion*, pp. 497–519. Chichester: Wiley.

Power, M.J. (2001). Memories of abuse and alien abduction: Close encounters of the therapeutic kind. In G.M. Davies and T. Dalgleish (eds.), *Recovered Memories: Seeking the Middle Ground*, pp. 247–261. Chichester: Wiley.

Power, M.J. (2005). Psychological approaches to bipolar disorders: A theoretical critique. *Clinical Psychology Review*, 25, 1101–1122.

Power, M.J. (2006). The structure of emotion: An empirical comparison of six models. *Cognition and Emotion*, 20, 694–713.

Power, M.J. (2010). *Emotion Focused Cognitive Therapy*. Chichester: Wiley-Blackwell.

Power, M.J. (2012). *Adieu to God: How Psychology Leads to Atheism*. Chichester: Wiley-Blackwell.

Power, M.J. (ed.) (2013). *The Wiley-Blackwell Handbook of Mood Disorders*, 2nd edn. Chichester: Wiley-Blackwell.

Power, M.J. (in press). *Happiness and Other Delusions*. Chichester: Wiley-Blackwell.

Power, M.J. and Dalgleish, T. (1997). *Cognition and Emotion: From Order to Disorder*. Hove: Psychology Press.

Power, M.J. and Dalgleish, T. (1999). Two routes to emotion: Some implications of multi-level theories of emotion for therapeutic practice. *Behavioural and Cognitive Psychotherapy*, 27, 129–141.

Power, M.J. and Dalgleish, T. (2008). *Cognition and Emotion: From Order to Disorder*, 2nd ed. Hove: Erlbaum.

Power, M.J. and Fyvie, C. (2013). The role of emotion in PTSD: Two preliminary studies. *Behavioural and Cognitive Psychotherapy*, 41, 162–172.

Power, M.J. and Tarsia, M. (2007). Basic and complex emotions in depression and anxiety. *Clinical Psychology and Psychotherapy*, 14, 19–31.

Power, M.J., de Jong, F., and Lloyd, A. (2002). The organisation of the self-concept in bipolar disorders: An empirical study and replication. *Cognitive Therapy and Research*, 26, 553–561.

Rachman, S.J. (2003). *The Treatment of Obsessions*. Oxford: Oxford University Press.

Rachman, S.J. (2004). *Anxiety*, 2nd edn. Hove: Psychology Press.

Read, J., Agar, K., Argyle, N., and Aderhold, V. (2003). Sexual and physical abuse during childhood and adulthood as predictors of hallucinations, delusions and thought disorder. *Psychology and Psychotherapy*, 76, 1–22.

Reuber, M. and Elger, C.E. (2003). Psychogenic nonepileptic seizures: Review and update. *Epilepsy and Behavior*, 4, 205–216.

Risch, N., Herrell, R., Lehner, T., et al. (2009). Interaction between the serotonin transporter gene (5-HTTLPR), stressful life events, and risk of depression: A meta-analysis. *Journal of the American Medical Association*, 301, 2462–2471.

Roediger, H.L. and McDermott, K.B. (1995). Creating false memories: Remembering words not presented in lists. *Journal of Experimental Psychology: Learning, Memory, and Cognition*, 21, 803–814.

Roelofs, K., Keijsers, G.P.J., Hoogduin, K.A.L., Naring, G.W.B., and Moene, F.C. (2002). Childhood abuse in patients with conversion disorder. *American Journal of Psychiatry*, 159, 1908–1913.

Rosaldo, M.Z. (1980). *Knowledge and Passion: Ilongot Notions of Self and Social Life*. Cambridge: Cambridge University Press.

Rosen, S.P. (2004). *War and Human Nature*. Princeton: Princeton University Press.

Rosenstein, D. and Oster, H. (1988). Differential facial responses to four basic tastes in new-borns. *Child Development*, 59, 1555–1568.

Ross, C.A. (1991). Epidemiology of multiple personality disorder and dissociation. *Psychiatric Clinics of North America*, 14, 503–517.

Ross, C.A., Joshi, S., and Currie, R. (1990). Dissociative experiences in the general population. *American Journal of Psychiatry*, 147, 1547–1552.

Rozin, P. and Fallon, A.E. (1987). A perspective on disgust. *Psychological Review*, 94, 23–41.

Russell, G. F.M. (1970). Anorexia nervosa: Its identity as an illness and its treatment. In J.H. Price (ed.), *Modern Trends in Psychological Medicine*, Vol. 2, pp. 131–164. London: Butterworths.

Russell, J. (1994). Is there universal recognition of emotion from facial expression? A review of the cross-cultural studies. *Psychological Bulletin*, 115, 102–141.

Russell, J.A. and Carroll, J.M. (1999). On the bipolarity of positive and negative affect. *Psychological Bulletin*, 125, 3–30.

Rutter, M. (1981). *Maternal Deprivation Reassessed*. London: Penguin.

Rutter, M. (1984). Psychopathology and development: 1. Childhood antecedents of adult psychiatric disorder. *Australian and New Zealand Journal of Psychiatry*, 18, 225–234.

Sanson, A., Hemphill, S.A., and Smart, D. (2004). Connections between temperament and social development: A review. *Social Development*, 13, 142–170.

Savino, A.C. and Fordtran, J.S. (2006). Factitious disease: Clinical lessons from case studies at Baylor University Medical Center. *Proceedings of Baylor University Medical Center*, 19, 195–208.

Schachter, S. and Singer, J.E. (1962). Cognitive, social, and physiological determinants of emotional state. *Psychological Review*, 69, 379–399.

Schmidt, U., Jiwany, A., and Treasure, J. (1993). A controlled study of alexithymia in eating disorders. *Comprehensive Psychiatry*, 34, 54–58.

Schmidt, N.B., Richey, J.A., Buckner, J.D., and Timpano, K.R. (2009). Attention training for generalized social anxiety disorder. *Journal of Abnormal Psychology*, 118, 5–14.

Schuster, J.P., Mouchabac, S., and LeStrat, Y. (2011). Hysterical mutism. *Encephale*, 37, 339–344.

Scull, A. (2011). *Madness: A Very Short Introduction*. Oxford: Oxford University Press.

Seligman, M. (1971). Phobias and preparedness. *Behavior Therapy*, 2, 307–320.

Shapira, N.A., Liu, H., He, A.G., et al. (2003). Brain-activation by disgust-inducing pictures in obsessive-compulsive disorder. *Biological Psychiatry*, 54, 751–756.

Shaver, P.R. and Hazan, C. (1988). A biased overview of the study of love. *Journal of Personal and Social Relationships*, 5, 474–501.

Shobe, K.K. and Schooler, J.W. (2001). Discovering fact and fiction: Case-based analyses of authentic and fabricated memories of abuse. In G.M. Davies and T. Dalgleish (eds.), *Recovered Memories: Seeking the Middle Ground*, pp. 95–151. Chichester: Wiley.

Shushan, G. (2009). *Conceptions of the Afterlife in Early Civilizations: Universalism, Constructivism and Near-Death Experience*. London: Continuum.

Sinkiewicz, A., Jaracz, M., Mackiewicz-Nartowicz, H., et al. (2013). Affective temperament in women with functional aphonia. *Journal of Voice*, 27, 129.e11–129.e14.

Smeets, F., Lataster, T., Dominguez, M., et al. (2010). Evidence that onset of psychosis in the population reflects early hallucinatory experiences that through environmental risks and affective dysregulation become complicated by delusions. *Schizophrenia Bulletin*, 38, 531–542.

Smolak, L. and Levine, M. P. (2007). Trauma, eating problems, and eating disorders. In S. Wonderlich, J.E. Mitchell, M. de Zwaan, and H. Sweiger (eds.), *Annual Review of Eating Disorders Part I—2007*, pp. 113–123. New York: Radcliff Publishing.

Spielberger, C.D., Gorsuch, R.L., and Lushene, R. (1970). *Trait Anxiety Scale*. Palo Alto, CA: Consulting Psychologists Press.

Spitzer, R.L. (1991). An outside-insider's views about revising the DSMs. *Journal of Abnormal Psychology*, 100, 294–296.

Stone, M., Laughren, T., Jones, M.L., et al. (2009). Risk of suicidality in clinical trials of anti-depressants in adults: analysis of proprietary data submitted to US Food and Drug Administration. *British Medical Journal*, 339, b2880.

Stroebe, W. and Stroebe, M.S. (1993). Determinants of adjustment to bereavement in younger widows and widowers. In M.S. Stroebe, W. Stroebe, and R.O. Hansson (eds.), *Handbook of Bereavement: Theory, Research, and Intervention*, pp. 208–226. Cambridge: Cambridge University Press.

Sturt, E. (1981). Hierarchical patterns in the distribution of psychiatric symptoms. *Psychological Medicine*, 11, 783–794.

Sun-Tzu (2002). *The Art of War*. London: Penguin.

Swainson, R., Hodges, J.R., Galton, C.J., Semple, J., Michael, A., and Dunn, B.D. (2001). Early detection and differential diagnosis of Alzheimer's disease and depression with neuropsychological tasks. *Dementia and Geriatric Cognitive Disorders*, 12, 265–280.

Tajfel, H. and Turner, J. (1979). An integrative theory of intergroup conflict. In W.G. Austin and S. Worchel (eds.), *The Social Psychology of Intergroup Relations* pp. 33–47. Monterey, CA: Brooks/Cole.

Tallis, F. (1995a). *Obsessive Compulsive Disorder: A Cognitive and Neuropsychological Perspective*. Chichester: Wiley.

Tallis, F. (1995b). The characteristics of obsessional thinking: Difficulty demonstrating the obvious? *Clinical Psychology and Psychotherapy*, 2, 24–39.

Tallis, F. (2004). *Love Sick: Love as a Mental Illness*. London: Century.

Tangney, J.P. (1999). The self-conscious emotions: Shame, guilt, embarrassment and pride. In T. Dalgleish and M.J. Power (eds.), *Handbook of Cognition and Emotion*, pp. 541–568. Chichester: Wiley.

Tantam, D. (2013). *Autism Spectrum Disorders Through the Life Span*. London: Jessica Kingsley.

Tay, L. and Diener, E. (2011). Needs and subjective well-being around the world. *Journal of Personality and Social Psychology*, 101, 354–365.

Taylor, S. (1999). *Anxiety Sensitivity: Theory, Research, and Treatment of the Fear of Anxiety*. Mahwah, NJ: Erlbaum.

Taylor, G.J., Bagby, R.M., and Parker, J.D.A. (1997). *Disorders of Affect Regulation: Alexithymia in Medical and Psychiatric Illness*. Cambridge: Cambridge University Press.

Teasdale, J.D. (1983). Negative thinking in depression: Cause, effect, or reciprocal relationship? *Advances in Behaviour Research and Therapy*, 5, 3–25.

Thomas, A., Chess, S., Birch, H.G., Hertzig, M., and Korn, S. (1963). *Behavioral Individuality in Early Childhood*. New York: New York University Press.

Tiihonen, J., Lonnqvist, J., Wahlbeck, K., Klaukka, T., Tanskanen, A., and Haukka, J. (2006). Antidepressants and the risk of suicide, attempted suicide, and overall mortality in a nation-wide cohort. *Archives of General Psychiatry*, 63, 1358–1367.

Tolin, D.F., Worhunsky, P., and Maltby, N. (2006). Are "obsessive" beliefs specific to OCD? A comparison across disorders. *Behaviour Research and Therapy*, 44, 469–480.

Tooby, J. and Cosmides, L. (1990). The past explains the present: Emotional adaptations and the structure of ancestral environments. *Ethology and Sociobiology*, 11, 375–424.

Tooby, J. and Cosmides, L. (1992). The psychological foundation of culture. In J.H. Barkow, L. Cosmides, and J. Tooby (eds.), *The Adapted Mind: Evolutionary Psychology and the Generation of Culture*, pp. 19–136. New York: Oxford University Press.

Treasure, J. and Schmidt, U. (2013). DBS for treatment-refractory anorexia nervosa. *The Lancet*, 381, 1338–1339.

Turner, T. (1995). Schizophrenia. In G. Berrios and R. Porter (eds.), *A History of Clinical Psychiatry*, pp. 349–359. London: Athlone Press.

Turner, T. (2003). *Scshizophrenia: Your Questions Answered*. Edinburgh: Churchill Livingstone.

Tutelyan, V.A., Chatterji, S., Baturin, A.K., Pogozheva, A.V., Kishko, O.N., and Akolzina, S.E. (2014). The Health and Functioning ICF-60 (HF-ICF-60): development and psychometric properties. *Clinical Psychology and Psychotherapy*. Epub ahead of print. doi: 10.1002/cpp.1909

Ussher, J.M. (2011). *The Madness of Women: Myth and Experience*. London: Routledge.

Van Egmond, M. and Jonker, D. (1988). Sexual abuse and physical assault: Risk factors for recurrent suicidal behaviour in women. *Tijdschraft die Psychiatrie*, 30, 21–38.

Vargas, L.A., Loye, F., and Hodde-Vargas, J. (1989). Exploring the multidimensional aspects of grief reactions. *American Journal of Psychiatry*, 146, 1484–1488.

Wall, P. (1999). *Pain: The Science of Suffering*. London: Weidenfeld and Nicolson.

Waller, G., Babbs, M., Milligan, R., Meyer, C., Ohanian, V., and Leung, N. (2003). Anger and core beliefs in the eating disorders. *International Journal of Eating Disorders*, 34, 118–124.

Watson, D. and Clark, L.A. (1992). Affects separable and inseparable: On the hierarchical arrangement of the negative affects. *Journal of Personality and Social Psychology*, 62, 489–505.

Watson, D. and Tellegen, A. (1999). Issues in dimensional structure of affect—effects of descriptors, measurement error, and response formats: Comment on Russell and Carroll (1999). *Psychological Bulletin*, 125, 601–610.

Watson, D., Clark, L.A., and Tellegen, A. (1988). Development and validation of brief measures of positive and negative affect: The PANAS scales. *Journal of Personality and Social Psychology*, 54, 1063–1070.

Watson, D., Weber, K., Assenheimer, J.S., Clark, L.A., Strauss, M.E., and McCormick, R.A. (1995a). Testing a tripartite model: 1. Evaluating the convergent and discriminant validity of anxiety and depression symptom scales. *Journal of Abnormal Psychology*, 104, 3–14.

Watson, D., Clark, L.A., Weber, K., Assenheimer, J.S., Strauss, M.E., and McCormick, R.A. (1995b). Testing a tripartite model: II. Exploring the symptom structure of anxiety and depression in student, adult, and patient samples. *Journal of Abnormal Psychology*, 104, 15–25.

Wegner, D.M. (1994). Ironic processes of mental control. *Psychological Review*, 101, 34–52.

Weinberger, D.A., Schwartz, G.E., and Davidson. R.J. (1979). Low-anxious, high anxious and repressive coping styles: Psychometric patterns and behavioural responses to stress. *Journal of Abnormal Psychology*, 88, 369–380.

Whitehead, W.E., Palsson, O., and Jones, K.R. (2002). Systematic review of the comorbidity of irritable bowel syndrome with other disorders: What are the causes and implications? *Gastroenterology*, 122, 1140–1156.

Whitehouse, A.J.O. and Bishop, D. (2009). Hemispheric division of function is the result of independent probabilistic biases. *Neuropsychologia*, 47, 1938–1943.

Widom, C.S. (1997). Child abuse, neglect, and witnessing violence. In D. Stoff, J. Breiling, and J. Maser (eds.), *Handbook of Antisocial Behavior*, pp. 159–170. New York: Wiley.

Wilkinson, T. (2010). *The Rise and Fall of Ancient Egypt*. London: Bloomsbury.

Wilkinson, R. and Pickett, K. (2010). *The Spirit Level: Why Equality is Better For Everyone*. London: Penguin.

Williams, L.M. (1995). Recovered memories of abuse in women with documented child sexual victimisation histories. *Journal of Traumatic Stress*, 8, 649–673.

Wimmer, H. and Perner, J. (1983). Beliefs about beliefs: representation and the containing function of wrong beliefs in young children's understanding of deception. *Cognition*, 13, 103–128.

Wing, L. (1981). Asperger's syndrome: A clinical account. *Psychological Medicine*, 11, 115–129.

Wing, L. (1991). The relationship between Asperger's syndrome and Kanner's autism. In U. Frith (ed.), *Autism and Asperger Syndrome*, pp. 93–121. Cambridge: Cambridge University Press.

Wing, J.K., Cooper, J.E., and Sartorius, N. (1974). *The Measurement and Classification of Psychiatric Symptoms*. Cambridge: Cambridge University Press.

Wolff, N.J., Darlington, A.E., Hunfeld, J.A.M., et al. (2011). The influence of attachment and temperament on venipuncture distress in 14-month-old infants: The Generation R study. *Infant Behavior and Development*, 34, 293–302.

Wolfgang, M.E. (1979). Aggression and violence: Crime and social control. In S. Feshback and A. Fraczek (eds.), *Aggression and Behavior Change*, pp. 139–157. New York: Praeger.

Wolfgang, M.E. and Ferracuti, F. (1967). *The Subculture of Violence*. New York: Barnes and Noble.

World Health Organization (1973). *Report of the International Pilot Study of Schizophrenia*, Vol. I. Geneva: World Health Organization.

World Health Organization (1992). *The ICD-10 Classification of Mental and Behavioural Disorders. Clinical Descriptions and Diagnostic Guidelines*. Geneva: World Health Organization.

World Health Organization (2001). *International Classification of Functioning, Disability and Health (ICF)*. Geneva: World Health Organization.

World Health Organization (2010). *World Malaria Report 2010*. Geneva: World Health Organization.

Wortman, C.B., Silver, R.C., and Kessler, R.C. (1993). The meaning of loss and adjustment to bereavement. In M.S. Stroebe, W. Stroebe, and R.O. Hansson (eds.), *Handbook of Bereavement: Theory, Research, and Intervention*, pp. 349–366. Cambridge: Cambridge University Press.

Wray, N.R., Pergadia, M.L., Blackwood, D.H., et al. (2010). Genome wide association study of major depressive disorder: New results, meta-analysis, and lessons learned. *Molecular Psychiatry*, 17, 36–48.

AUTHOR INDEX

SUBJECT INDEX